A Summary of the February 2010
Forum on the Future of Nursing

EDUCATION

Committee on the Robert Wood Johnson
Foundation Initiative on the Future of Nursing,
at the Institute of Medicine

INSTITUTE OF MEDICINE
OF THE NATIONAL ACADEMIES

THE NATIONAL ACADEMIES PRESS
Washington, D.C.
www.nap.edu

THE NATIONAL ACADEMIES PRESS • 500 Fifth Street, N.W. • Washington, DC 20001

NOTICE: The project that is the subject of this report was approved by the Governing Board of the National Research Council, whose members are drawn from the councils of the National Academy of Sciences, the National Academy of Engineering, and the Institute of Medicine. The members of the committee responsible for the report were chosen for their special competences and with regard for appropriate balance.

Support for this project was provided by the Robert Wood Johnson Foundation (Contract No. 65815). Any opinions, findings, conclusions, or recommendations expressed in this publication are those of the author(s) and do not necessarily reflect the views of the organizations or agencies that provided support for the project.

International Standard Book Number-13: 978-0-309-15282-2
International Standard Book Number-10: 0-309-15282-8

Additional copies of this report are available from the National Academies Press, 500 Fifth Street, N.W., Lockbox 285, Washington, DC 20055; (800) 624-6242 or (202) 334-3313 (in the Washington metropolitan area); Internet, http://www.nap.edu.

For more information about the Institute of Medicine, visit the IOM home page at: **www.iom.edu.**

Cover credit: Photos by Sam Kittner/kittner.com.

Suggested citation: IOM (Institute of Medicine). 2010. *A summary of the February 2010 forum on the future of nursing: Education.* Washington, DC: The National Academies Press.

"Knowing is not enough; we must apply.
Willing is not enough; we must do."
—Goethe

INSTITUTE OF MEDICINE
OF THE NATIONAL ACADEMIES

Advising the Nation. Improving Health.

THE NATIONAL ACADEMIES
Advisers to the Nation on Science, Engineering, and Medicine

The **National Academy of Sciences** is a private, nonprofit, self-perpetuating society of distinguished scholars engaged in scientific and engineering research, dedicated to the furtherance of science and technology and to their use for the general welfare. Upon the authority of the charter granted to it by the Congress in 1863, the Academy has a mandate that requires it to advise the federal government on scientific and technical matters. Dr. Ralph J. Cicerone is president of the National Academy of Sciences.

The **National Academy of Engineering** was established in 1964, under the charter of the National Academy of Sciences, as a parallel organization of outstanding engineers. It is autonomous in its administration and in the selection of its members, sharing with the National Academy of Sciences the responsibility for advising the federal government. The National Academy of Engineering also sponsors engineering programs aimed at meeting national needs, encourages education and research, and recognizes the superior achievements of engineers. Dr. Charles M. Vest is president of the National Academy of Engineering.

The **Institute of Medicine** was established in 1970 by the National Academy of Sciences to secure the services of eminent members of appropriate professions in the examination of policy matters pertaining to the health of the public. The Institute acts under the responsibility given to the National Academy of Sciences by its congressional charter to be an adviser to the federal government and, upon its own initiative, to identify issues of medical care, research, and education. Dr. Harvey V. Fineberg is president of the Institute of Medicine.

The **National Research Council** was organized by the National Academy of Sciences in 1916 to associate the broad community of science and technology with the Academy's purposes of furthering knowledge and advising the federal government. Functioning in accordance with general policies determined by the Academy, the Council has become the principal operating agency of both the National Academy of Sciences and the National Academy of Engineering in providing services to the government, the public, and the scientific and engineering communities. The Council is administered jointly by both Academies and the Institute of Medicine. Dr. Ralph J. Cicerone and Dr. Charles M. Vest are chair and vice chair, respectively, of the National Research Council.

www.national-academies.org

COMMITTEE ON THE ROBERT WOOD JOHNSON FOUNDATION INITIATIVE ON THE FUTURE OF NURSING, AT THE INSTITUTE OF MEDICINE

DONNA E. SHALALA (*Chair*), University of Miami, Coral Gables, FL
LINDA BURNES BOLTON (*Vice Chair*), Cedars-Sinai Health System and Research Institute, Los Angeles, CA
MICHAEL BLEICH, Oregon Health & Science University School of Nursing, Portland
TROYEN A. BRENNAN, CVS Caremark, Woonsocket, RI
ROBERT E. CAMPBELL, Johnson & Johnson (*retired*), New Brunswick, NJ
LEAH DEVLIN, University of North Carolina at Chapel Hill, School of Public Health
CATHERINE DOWER, University of California–San Francisco
ROSA GONZALEZ-GUARDA, University of Miami, Coral Gables, FL
DAVID C. GOODMAN, Dartmouth Medical School, Hanover, NH
JENNIE CHIN HANSEN, AARP, Washington, DC
C. MARTIN HARRIS, Cleveland Clinic, Cleveland, OH
ANJLI AURORA HINMAN, Intown Midwifery, Atlanta, GA
WILLIAM D. NOVELLI, Georgetown University, Washington, DC
LIANA ORSOLINI-HAIN, City College of San Francisco, CA
YOLANDA PARTIDA, University of California–San Francisco, Fresno
ROBERT D. REISCHAUER, Urban Institute, Washington, DC
JOHN W. ROWE, Columbia University, New York
BRUCE C. VLADECK, Nexera Consulting, New York

Study Staff
JUDITH A. SALERNO, Executive Officer
SUSAN HASSMILLER, Director, Robert Wood Johnson Foundation Initiative on the Future of Nursing, at the Institute of Medicine
ADRIENNE STITH BUTLER, Senior Program Officer
ANDREA M. SCHULTZ, Associate Program Officer
KATHARINE BOTHNER, Research Associate
THELMA L. COX, Administrative Assistant
TONIA E. DICKERSON, Senior Program Assistant
GINA IVEY, Communications Director, Robert Wood Johnson Foundation Initiative on the Future of Nursing, at the Institute of Medicine

LORI MELICHAR, Research Director, Robert Wood Johnson Foundation Initiative on the Future of Nursing, at the Institute of Medicine
JULIE FAIRMAN, Nurse Scholar-in-Residence

Consultants
PAUL LIGHT, New York University
STEVE OLSON, Technical Writer

Reviewers

This report has been reviewed in draft form by individuals chosen for their diverse perspectives and technical expertise, in accordance with procedures approved by the National Research Council's Report Review Committee. The purpose of this independent review is to provide candid and critical comments that will assist the institution in making its published report as sound as possible and to ensure that the report meets institutional standards for objectivity, evidence, and responsiveness to the study charge. The review comments and draft manuscript remain confidential to protect the integrity of the process. We wish to thank the following individuals for their review of this report:

Sr. Rosemary Donley, Duquesne University School of Nursing
Greer Glazer, College of Nursing and Health Sciences, University of Massachusetts–Boston
Hugh H. Tilson, University of North Carolina at Chapel Hill, School of Public Health
Rachael Watman, John A. Hartford Foundation

Although the reviewers listed above have provided many constructive comments and suggestions, they were not asked to endorse the final draft of the report before its release. The review of this report was overseen by **Ada Sue Hinshaw,** Graduate School of Nursing, Uniformed Services University of the Health Sciences. Appointed by the National Research Council and the Institute of Medicine, she was responsible for making certain that an independent examination of this report was carried out in accordance with institutional procedures and that all review comments were carefully considered. Responsibility for the final content of this report rests entirely with the authors and the institution.

Preface

The Initiative on the Future of Nursing, a collaborative effort of the Robert Wood Johnson Foundation (RWJF) and the Institute of Medicine (IOM), took place during a pivotal period in the history of health care in the United States. From the beginning of the 2-year initiative, the national conversation was dominated by the effort to achieve meaningful reforms in its health care system, culminating with President Barack Obama signing the *Patient Protection and Affordable Care Act* into law on March 23, 2010. It was a fascinating time to serve as members of the IOM committee that was charged with developing a set of action-oriented recommendations for the future of nursing—the profession that makes up the single largest component of the health care system.

On February 22, 2010, just a month before that historic day in health care reform, the Initiative on the Future of Nursing held the last public forum in a series of three at the University of Texas MD Anderson Cancer Center. This forum, which covered the education of nurses, consisted of three armchair discussions. Each discussion was led by a moderator from the committee and focused on three broad, overlapping subjects: what to teach, how to teach, and where to teach. The verbal exchange among the discussants and moderators, prompted by additional questions from committee members at the forum, produced a wide-ranging and informative examination of questions that are critical to the future of nursing education. Additionally, testimony presented by 12 individuals and comments made by members of the audience during an open-microphone session provided the committee with valuable input from a range of perspectives.

Several important messages flowed from the forum discussions, including:

- The new basics in nursing education are collaboration within the profession and across other health professions, communication, and systems thinking;
- Nurses, particularly nurse educators, need to keep up with a rapidly changing knowledge base and new technologies throughout their careers to ensure a well-educated workforce;
- Care for older adults, increasingly occurring outside of acute care settings, will be a large and growing component of nursing in the future, and the nursing education system needs to prepare educators and practitioners for that reality;
- The nation will face serious consequences if the number of nursing educators is not adequate to develop a more diverse nursing workforce adequate in both number and competencies to meet the needs of diverse populations across the lifespan;
- Technology—such as that used in high-fidelity simulations—that fosters problem-solving and critical-thinking skills in nurses will be essential for nursing education to produce sufficient numbers of competent, well-educated nurses;
- Resources and partnerships available in the community should be used to prepare nurses who can serve their communities;
- Articulation agreements and education consortiums among different kinds of institutions can provide multiple entry points and continued opportunities for progression through an educational and career ladder; and
- In addition to necessary skill sets, nursing education needs to provide students with the ability to mature as professionals and to continue learning throughout their careers.

While the health care legislation signed into law in March is momentous, the discussions leading up to the legislation were marked by a notable deficiency. The voices of nurses did not play a prominent role in the debate over health care reform, even though nurses are central to the delivery of high-quality, safe, effective care. The Initiative on the Future of Nursing has provided an opportunity for the perspective of nurses and other stakeholders to enter the ongoing discussion about the future of the profession and how it should play a role in ensuring the health of Americans.

As the U.S. health care system continues to evolve, the role of nurses also needs to evolve. Nurses must strike a delicate balance among advancing science, translating and applying research, and caring for individuals and families across all settings. Preparing nurses to achieve this balance is a significant challenge. The education system should ensure that nurses have the intellectual capacity, human responsiveness, flexibility, and leadership skills to provide care and promote health whenever and wherever needed. Education leaders and faculty need to prepare nurses with the competencies they need now and in the future. They need to prepare nurses to work and assume leadership roles not just in hospitals, but in communities, clinics, homes, and everywhere else nurses are needed.

As Dr. John R. Lumpkin, senior vice president and director of the Health Care Group at RWJF, said during his introduction to the forum, nurses must be involved in planning, carrying out, and leading changes in the health care system. The committee's job is to figure out how to make that imperative a reality.

Donna E. Shalala
Committee Chair

Michael Bleich
Committee Member
and Forum Planning Group Chair

Acknowledgments

The Robert Wood Johnson Foundation (RWJF) Initiative on the Future of Nursing, at the Institute of Medicine, wishes to thank all those who contributed to the success of the *Forum on the Future of Nursing: Education*. The forum was graciously hosted by the University of Texas MD Anderson Cancer Center; its staff, particularly Cheryl Franklin, Lisa Green, Demetria Marks, Barbara Summers, and Cherie Wade, provided valuable support throughout the planning process and the forum.

The Initiative would like to thank the speakers, panelists, and all who provided testimony at the forum; the insight and experience that was shared greatly contributed to the committee's deliberations. The Initiative would also like to recognize the alumni from various RWJF fellow and scholar programs who participated in the forum. These individuals met to reflect on the day's discussions and offered the committee several innovative ideas to consider for the future of nursing education.

While in Houston, the Initiative had the opportunity to visit a number of nearby education and training programs for nurses and other professionals. The Initiative would like to express gratitude to the following individuals, and their colleagues, for warmly welcoming us into their learning communities: Ann Coleman, Karen Lyon, and Kelly Vandenberg at Texas Woman's University; Jenny Knotts, Debbie Nguyen, and Lori Wheaton at the National Aeronautics and Space Administration; and Patricia Starck and Michelle Thomas at the University of Texas Health Science Center at Houston School of Nursing.

The forum planning group, chaired by Michael Bleich, skillfully shaped the day's events. The group included Troy Brennan, Linda Burnes Bolton, Jennie Chin Hansen, David Goodman,

Anjli Aurora Hinman, Liana Orsolini-Hain, Donna E. Shalala, and Bruce Vladeck.

For their steadfast and creative work throughout the course of the forum, we would like to recognize the Initiative staff members, led by Susan Hassmiller and Adrienne Stith Butler, with guidance and oversight from Judith Salerno. The following individuals were involved in planning the forum, day-of support, and production of this summary: Katharine Bothner, Thelma Cox, Julie Dashiell, Tonia Dickerson, Gina Ivey, Lori Melichar, Abbey Meltzer, and Andrea Schultz. The forum was webcast by ON24 and transcribed by Joy Biletz. The Initiative is grateful to Steve Olson for his editorial and writing assistance, Laura Penny for copyediting the summary, and Dan Banks for designing the cover. We would also like to recognize the contributions of the following staff and consultants to this activity: Clyde Behney, Christie Bell, Julie Fairman, Christine Gorman, Amy Levey, Paul Light, Tamara Parr, Sharon Reis, Christine Stencel, Vilija Teel, Lauren Tobias, Jackie Turner, Gary Walker, and Jordan Wyndelts.

Finally, the Initiative would like to express its appreciation to RWJF, whose generous financial support, and mission to improve the health and health care of all Americans, made the forum possible.

Contents

APPENDIXES

1

Introduction

On February 22, 2010, the Robert Wood Johnson Foundation (RWJF) Initiative on the Future of Nursing, at the Institute of Medicine (IOM), held a forum on the future of nursing at the University of Texas MD Anderson Cancer Center in Houston. This forum was designed to examine challenges and opportunities associated with nursing education overall. The forum was the last of three that were convened to gather information and discuss ideas related to the future of nursing. The first forum, held on October 19, 2009, at Cedars-Sinai Medical Center in Los Angeles, focused on the future of nursing in acute care. The second forum, on December 3, 2009, at the Community College of Philadelphia, examined the future of nursing care in the community, with emphases on community health, public health, primary care, and long-term care.

The forums have been part of an intensive information-gathering effort by an IOM committee that is the cornerstone of the Initiative on the Future of Nursing. The committee will use the information collected at these forums, at its two technical workshops, from data provided by the RWJF Nursing Research Network, and from a number of commissioned papers to inform the development of its findings, conclusions, and recommendations. The committee's final recommendations will be presented in a report in fall 2010 on the capacity of the nursing workforce to meet the demands of the changing health care system.

Each of the three forums was planned with the guidance of a small group of committee members; the planning group for this forum was led by Dr. Michael Bleich. The half-day forums were not meant to be an exhaustive examination of all settings where nurses practice nor an exhaustive examination of the complexity of the nursing profession as a whole. Given the limited amount of time for each forum, a comprehensive review of all facets and all players of each of the main forum themes was not possible. Rather, the forums were meant to inform the committee on important topics within the nursing profession and highlight some of the key challenges, barriers, opportunities, and innovations that nurses face while working in an evolving health care system. Many of the critical challenges, barriers, opportunities, and innovations discussed at the forums overlap across settings and throughout the nursing profession and also apply to other providers and individuals who work with nurses.

Unlike the two previous forums, which featured a series of presentations, the Houston forum was organized into three armchair discussions that were moderated by members of the IOM committee. The first discussion, moderated by Dr. Michael Bleich, examined the broad topic of what to teach and the ideal future state of nursing curriculums (Chapter 2). The second, "How to Teach" (Chapter 3), focused on methodologies and strategies, as well as partnerships and collaboratives, that could be used for educating nurses and was moderated by Dr. Linda Burnes Bolton. The third, "Where to Teach" (Chapter 4), was moderated by Jennie Chin Hansen and dealt with various venues and locations where nurses could be educated. This summary of the forum describes the main points made during the discussions. It also summarizes the oral testimony presented by 12 forum attendees, along with remarks made during an open-microphone session at the end of the forum (Chapter 5). A complete agenda of the forum can be found in Appendix B, and biosketches of the discussants and moderators can be found in Appendix C. The remaining sections of this chapter describe two activities that occurred in conjunction with the forum and present the welcoming remarks of Dr. John R. Lumpkin of RWJF and Dr. John R. Mendelsohn of the University of Texas MD Anderson Cancer Center.

Comments made at the forum should not be interpreted as positions of the IOM committee, RWJF, the IOM, or the University of Texas MD Anderson Cancer Center. Committee members' questions and comments do not necessarily reflect their personal views or the conclusions that will be in the committee's report. However, the questions and comments were designed to elicit information and perspectives to help guide the committee's deliberations.

SITE VISITS

Following the forum, committee members participated in visits to one of three sites in Houston: the University of Texas Health (UTH) Science Center at Houston School of Nursing, Texas Woman's University (TWU), or the National Aeronautics and Space Administration (NASA). Detailed observations made during these site visits are not part of this summary, but the site visits have informed the committee's deliberations on nursing education.

During the site visits, committee members had the opportunity to talk with nursing students, educators, administrators, and experts in training for quality, safety, and collaboration about some of the innovations being used. The site visit at UTH included demonstrations in a physical assessment lab using retired physicians as educators, a high-fidelity simulation lab, and a nurse-managed clinic. This visit also included discussion of educational models such as distance learning and accelerated doctoral programs. Those who visited TWU saw a demonstration in a high-fidelity simulation lab and heard discussion of technology use in educational settings and interdisciplinary education programs. The site visit to NASA focused on training for quality and safety, collaboration in a team environment, and continuing education. Participants at this site visit heard discussions about resource management and strategies for error reduction through collaboration.

ROBERT WOOD JOHNSON FOUNDATION SOLUTIONS SESSION

Following the site visits, a select group of RWJF scholars and fellows[1] hosted by RWJF met to discuss what they heard at the forum and observed on the site visits in the context of their own expertise, knowledge, and judgment. This session was independent of the IOM committee and the forum on the future of nursing. The goal of this session was to

---

[1]RWJF works to build human capital by supporting individuals who seek to advance health and health care in America. RWJF invited alumni of 17 of its scholar, fellow, and leader programs to participate in the Forum on the Future of Nursing. The alumni came from a variety of backgrounds and disciplines, including academia, service delivery, research, policy, and health plan administration. Many participants were alumni of the RWJF Executive Nurse Fellows Program and the RWJF Nurse Faculty Scholars Program. Non-nurse participants included alumni of the Investigator Award Program, the RWJF Health Policy Fellows Program, and the RWJF Clinical Scholar Program.

provide an opportunity for the fellows and scholars to consider solutions and the most promising directions for nursing education.

The solutions offered by the fellows and scholars are not described in this summary of the forum. But summaries of their solutions were provided to the committee for its review and consideration.

WELCOMING REMARKS

Dr. John R. Lumpkin, senior vice president and director of the Health Care Group at RWJF, noted that the mission of RWJF is to improve the health and health care of all Americans. The Foundation's mission has placed it at the center of a critically important period in U.S. history, he said. At the time of the forum, shortly before the passage of health care reform, 46 million Americans were uninsured (DeNavas-Walt et al., 2009). The cost of health care was continuing to rise, and many health care providers were increasingly dissatisfied with their work environment—so much so that many were thinking about leaving the field, he said. "Regardless of what happens in Washington this year, the status quo in health and health care is unsustainable," he said. "Change is in the wind."

Nurses are the largest component of the health care system. Not only do nurses need to be involved in changing the system in which they work, Lumpkin said, but "nurses have to help lead the change." The IOM committee's task is to examine how that change will happen and the role that nurses will play in the process. The Initiative hosted these three forums to give nurses and other health care providers a voice in the committee's deliberations. At the same time, the Foundation is committed to the work that will need to be done after the committee has released its report: the committee's recommendations will need to be implemented "so that nursing and nurses can play their rightful role in effecting the change that is going to be so important for the future of this country," said Lumpkin.

Dr. John Mendelsohn, president of the University of Texas MD Anderson Cancer Center, also welcomed the committee, the more than 300 people who attended the forum, and the additional 330 who registered for the forum's live webcast. The Cancer Center has 3,900 registered nurses and 50 licensed vocational nurses, Mendelsohn said. Of the registered nurses, 600 have master's degrees, and more than 20 have doctoral degrees. In 2010, the center will see more than 100,000 cancer patients, with 33,000 new registrants, and will place 11,000 patients in therapeutic clinical trials, he said.

Education is "one of the four pillars of our mission. The others are patient care, research, and prevention," Mendelsohn explained. The Cancer Center has an academic department of nursing that is devoted to nursing research and teaching. It also offers every nurse, at every level, an opportunity to advance their practices, careers, and goals. "We are grateful to have the resources to make nursing education and advancement a priority. We know that this makes a difference in every facet of our patient care, research, and institutional culture," he said. The work of the IOM committee will be an important response to the challenge of improving the quality and efficiency of U.S. health care, Mendelsohn said.

2

What to Teach

Throughout the discussions at the three forums on the future of nursing, members of the Institute of Medicine (IOM) committee heard informative evidence and memorable and insightful observations about the scope of nursing's contributions to the delivery of care and the advancement of science, said Dr. Michael Bleich, dean, and Dr. Carol A. Lindeman, Distinguished Professor for the School of Nursing at Oregon Health & Science University. Nursing education is the foundation for nurses' ability to assume a variety of challenging roles throughout the health care system. The preparation of nurses "requires a great deal of intelligence, integrity, and focus," Bleich said.

As moderator of the first armchair discussion, which considered the topic "What to Teach," Bleich focused the discussion on the educational needs at both basic and advanced levels to ensure a well-educated, competent workforce. He led an engaging and interactive discussion with four prominent leaders in nursing education: Dr. Linda Cronenwett, professor and dean emeritus for the School of Nursing at the University of North Carolina–Chapel Hill; Dr. Terry Fulmer, Erline Perkins McGriff Professor and dean of the College of Nursing at New York University; Dr. Marla Salmon, Robert G. and Jean A. Reid Dean in Nursing and professor in the School of Nursing at the University of Washington; and Dr. M. Elaine Tagliareni, chief program officer for the National League of Nursing and former professor of nursing and Independence Foundation chair in Community Health Nursing Education at the Community College of Philadelphia. The discussion touched on many concerns and areas of opportunity to improve nursing education.

Bleich opened the conversation by asking the four expert discussants what every nurse's education should include: "What is the knowledge needed to ensure a competent practitioner?" He continued by asking about the knowledge needed in a range of advanced nursing roles: "How do you see the roles and the education essential for preparing competent nurse specialists evolving?" Bleich also asked discussants to provide key recommendations they would like the committee to consider as it concludes its deliberations and develops the recommendations for its final report.

BASIC NURSING EDUCATION

As the largest component of the health care workforce, nurses play a vital role in delivering care across a wide range of settings: from acute care and long-term care facilities, to public health and community health clinics, to schools and homes, and everywhere in between. In addition to delivering care, nurses also fill leadership and advisory positions and serve as researchers, scientists, and educators. As Bleich said in his introductory remarks, education gives nurses the ability to fill these positions; basic education is particularly important because it provides the foundation on which everything else is built.

Salmon highlighted four realities that are driving changes in nursing education: more nurses are working outside of hospitals as care shifts formally and informally into communities; evidence that could inform practice is growing rapidly, but is not well integrated into either education or practice; the need for nurses to effectively work in and lead teams is increasing; and numbers alone will not fill the widening gap between the supply of nurses and the growing need for their services—additional research and new knowledge will be required. Tagliareni added that changes in patient demographics, care needs, and job demands have produced a need for changes in the nursing curriculum, particularly at the basic education level.

Building a Strong Foundation

Nursing education needs to provide all students with the scientific background, practice-based knowledge, clinical reasoning skills, and ethical comportment to enter the practice of nursing, said Cronenwett. To better prepare students with the necessary scientific background, curriculums would benefit from the creation of a common base of prerequisites.

Additionally, educators should work to improve the links among knowledge, practice, and clinical reasoning skills in courses, Cronenwett said.

The approach to the basic curriculum is currently "siloed"; this approach may limit the ability of graduates to understand, manage, and make judgments in complex emerging care environments and community-based practice, Tagliareni said. Today, nursing education focuses on patient–nurse interactions, but to improve quality of care, nurses also need to think in terms of health care systems. They need to understand quality and safety issues, the importance of team approaches to problem solving, and the need for patient education.

The nursing pedagogy needs to be linked with the dissemination of knowledge, Tagliareni said. Nursing education needs to move away from the "additive curriculum" toward a curriculum that emphasizes competent performance through active learning. In addition, Salmon said students need to learn how to assess, use, and manage knowledge so they can access it when needed instead of being something they "cram into their heads" during the learning process.

Once nurses have entered the profession, they need to further develop their knowledge in relation to specific settings, patient or community populations, and care teams, Cronenwett asserted. Having a strong foundation in these key areas will better prepare nurses to acquire this additional knowledge throughout their careers. To improve the transition to practice, she suggested a mandated, postlicensure transition-to-practice residency program that would facilitate continued learning and increase the depth of knowledge needed to practice.

Educating to Meet the Health Needs of Americans

Basic nursing education needs to reflect the new world that is taking shape and the changes in U.S. patient populations, Tagliareni and Fulmer emphasized. The demographics of the American population are shifting; the population is aging and becoming more diverse. The way health care is provided is also shifting; care frequently requires a team of providers working together across settings.

Fulmer said the health care system is moving from an urgent situation to a crisis, given that the population of people over 65 will double over the next 20 years, with an additional 10 million more people over the age of 80 by then. Older adults account for 35 percent of all hospital stays, 34 percent of all prescriptions, 38 percent of all emergency medical responses, and 90 percent of all nursing home use (IOM, 2008). Basic nursing education needs to cover topics such as geriatric syndromes, sleep disorders, dementia, delirium, depression, and chronic care management. "This is highly complex nursing," Fulmer explained. Tagliareni added that when educating students, care for older adults should be the prototype used for the future of nursing. Such care involves assessment of function and expectations, health promotion and self-care, chronic care management, life transitions, and the promotion of human productivity despite loss and frailty.

Interdisciplinary team skills and collaboration will be essential for coping with the complexity of care for an older population and to ensure that patients receive continuous care across settings and providers. Nurses need to know how to work with patient care attendants, with physicians, and with specialists across teams under a variety of circumstances. Salmon said nurses have never been able to "go it alone," which means that basic nursing education must prepare graduates to work in teams. Nurses need to be able to lead effectively across settings and within groups, she said. Fulmer noted that simulations could be particularly valuable in conveying this type of knowledge.

Basic nursing education also needs to devote more effort to fostering diversity, including culturally sensitive and relationship-centered care, Tagliareni said. Institutionalizing a commitment to diversity has posed substantial challenges in education institutes, but it also has led to powerful examples of faculty creating innovative models that tackle issues of inclusion, justice, and diversity in a world that is increasingly without borders, she said.

Educating for Continuous Improvement

Nursing education needs to prepare graduates who understand that part of the daily work of nurses is to continuously improve the delivery of nursing care and health care in local settings, Cronenwett said. Graduates need the competencies and skills required to participate in and lead quality improvement efforts wherever they practice. "Those two things are very important—how to do the work, and how to improve the work," she noted.

Both the IOM and the Robert Wood Johnson Foundation have devoted considerable attention to problems with quality and safety in health care, Cronenwett pointed out. Nurses should be able to help solve these problems by working with empowered patients, collaborating in a team environment, being familiar with the tools of quality improvement, understanding cultures of safety, and knowing how to use informatics to enhance the reliability of care, she concluded.

A Spirit of Inquiry and Life-Long Learning

Students need to learn the fundamentals of their profession, but they also need to develop a "spirit of inquiry," Tagliareni said. This spirit of inquiry will allow nurses to examine the evidence that underlies clinical nursing practice, learn to access research evidence, question underlying assumptions, and offer new insights to improve the quality of care for patients, families, and communities.

Nurses need to be encouraged and engaged to continue life-long learning in formal ways, Bleich asserted. Such learning can occur on topics such as collaboration, team work, and health systems. "[Nurses] need to be engaged in a commitment to and a passion for education in all its various forms," Bleich said. Salmon added that initial education for nurses is just that—education needs to continue over time. Additionally, people intending to become nurses should see the profession as "a calling, a commitment, and an intellectual adventure," she said.

Future Directions for Basic Education

As requested by Bleich, each discussant offered recommendations to the committee about necessary actions to improve basic nursing education. According to Cronenwett, scholarships, loan forgiveness programs, and institutional capacity awards could increase the number and proportion of newly licensed nurses graduating from baccalaureate and higher degree programs, which would produce more prelicensure graduates who would be more likely to go on to graduate school.

Tagliareni said basic nursing education should refocus on the fundamentals to reflect the expanded settings of care. "What is fundamental may not be accomplished by running students through subspecialties," such as obstetrics and pediatrics, she said. Basic nursing education also should rethink approaches to safety, patient-centered care, cultural competence, and clinical judgment.

Fulmer emphasized that nursing schools should teach all students about geriatric syndromes, chronic care management, team skills, collaboration, and communication.

Salmon said nursing schools need to develop knowledge management, access, and use of tools and strategies rather than burdening students with information that is hardwired into the curriculum. "What we ought to be hardwiring is the ability to manage and use knowledge in real time in both education and practice," she said.

ADVANCED NURSING EDUCATION

Beyond basic education, advanced nursing education is critical to the profession for several reasons, Bleich said. It prepares nurses for a variety of specialized advanced practice roles that are essential in the health care system; these advanced roles include nurse practitioners, clinical nurse specialists, certified registered nurse anesthetists, and certified nurse midwives. It produces the nurse educators who will prepare future generations of nurses, and it equips nurses to do research to advance care, including research done as members of interdisciplinary teams of health care experts.

The Pipeline

In the next 10 years, Fulmer noted, more than 40 percent of registered nurses will approach retirement age, creating a large gap in the workforce at all levels of education (Buerhaus et al., 2000). Tagliareni expressed concern about the low number of prelicensure students who are progressing to the advanced practice role. "We are not moving them in the numbers that we need in order to develop those roles both in practice and certainly for nurse educators," she said. Cronenwett said the number of people getting master's and doctoral degrees in nursing is unlikely to rise appreciably until more people come into nursing through universities. "That is overwhelmingly the group of people who go on," she said. A state-by-state commitment is needed to increase the percentage of people who are exposed to nursing in universities, she added.

To prepare future generations of nurses and move students to higher levels of education, the education system requires an adequate number of well-prepared faculty. More focus is needed on the specialized role of nurse educators and on the preparation and development of faculty, Tagliareni said. Faculty need to understand the best practices and strategies in learning and teaching to ensure the development of critical thinking skills in their students. Nursing schools and programs need to place additional emphasis on faculty recruitment and retention strategies, Tagliareni added.

Advanced Curriculums and Competencies

Current advanced practice curriculums provide only limited exposure to information about how to achieve change and how to evaluate the impact on quality when evidence-based solutions are adopted, Tagliareni said. Advanced practice nurses (APRNs)[1] need these important tools, as well as critical thinking skills to optimize patient care. Obtaining and applying necessary skills and knowledge to implement and evaluate change requires education in a wide portfolio of topics, new pedagogies, and graduate-level competencies.

APRNs will be increasingly responsible for primary care; already, there are nearly 600 million patient visits to nurse practitioners each year (AANP, 2010). APRNs need to be able to deal with the complexity of not just a disease or disorder, but also the care environment, including multiple specialists and disciplines, Fulmer said. To manage this complexity, teaching about teamwork and collaboration "has to be in every single class." In addition to competencies for primary care, the aging of the population will require nurses, especially APRNs, to have competencies to ensure quality care outcomes for older adults, Fulmer explained.

Salmon called for a distinction to be made between what nurses need to learn as they prepare to enter practice and what information and knowledge is needed to continue their practice across their career. Too much knowledge is compressed into advanced degree programs, she noted. The pharmacy profession, for example, has realized that memorizing all drug interactions is impossible because so many exist. Instead, practitioners access drug interaction databases so that "you use that knowledge when you need it," Salmon said. This strategy could greatly benefit the nursing profession.

---

[1]APRNs meet additional requirements in education and clinical practice, generally a master's degree or another form of advanced clinical preparation. APRNs include nurse practitioners, nurse anesthetists, nurse midwives, and clinical nurse specialists.

Once nurses reach the advanced practice level, they need to be able to ensure their own professional development and that of others, demonstrate leadership, and promote positive change in people and systems. "[APRNs] are change agents . . . for both personal and professional growth of themselves and others, and we count on them for direction," Tagliareni said. As with basic nursing education, taking on this role requires an understanding of the health care system as a whole.

APRNs and Nurse Specialists

Society needs APRNs now and will continue to need them in increasing numbers in the future. Evidence demonstrates that master's degree specialist programs are preparing competent nurse practitioners, midwives, anesthetists, nurse managers, and other APRNs, Cronenwett said. Additionally, a good alignment is in place among the requirements for licensure, certification, education, and accreditation, and this alignment should not be disrupted, she said.

Cronenwett further asserted that advanced practice should not require the attainment of a doctoral degree as the entry to advanced practice. She expressed concern that requiring a doctoral degree would diminish the number of advanced practice graduates per year and increase the costs to students and society to produce APRNs.

Individuals should make choices about the kind of doctorate they want to pursue after they know more about nursing and about the kinds of roles they want to fill within the profession, Cronenwett said. Nurses also should make these choices once they are competent practitioners and thus capable of developing the doctoral-level skills and knowledge (through the D.N.P. or Ph.D.) to have greater impact on practice, science, health policy, leadership, and the improvement of health care, she said.

Improving Practice Through Research

"The gap between the need for care and the availability of nurses will only continue to grow, and this gap cannot be filled through numbers alone," said Salmon. "For nurses to improve access to and the quality and cost of care, new knowledge needs to be developed." While other health disciplines, such as medicine and pharmacy, have a strong, well-funded research foundation, nursing has not experienced the same level of support or engagement, she said.

Federal funding for nursing research is insufficient to meet the challenges of advancing care for the future, Salmon said. Of the more than $30 billion the National Institutes of Health spends on research, only about $145 million is committed to nursing research through the National Institute of Nursing Research (NIH Office of Budget, 2010). "That is paltry," she said, and indicates a devaluing or inattention to the development of the science as a foundation for nursing.

"Lack of funding and support for training nurse scientists poses a significant threat to the future of care; additionally, the underpinnings of care and research around care [are] being eroded," Salmon said. Nurse scientists often carry significant financial burdens, which ultimately affect their career trajectories and contributions to research. Predoctoral nursing students generally do not earn a living wage, she said, which results in the need for students to make money while pursuing graduate education and to find ways to pay off debt after completion of their degrees. With an average age of completion of 46 (compared to 33 in other disciplines) for a nurse Ph.D. and heavy loan burdens, nurse scholars often forego important postdoctoral training and make career choices that may divert their focus on science, she said (Berlin and Sechrist, 2002). The net result is that nurse scholars have significantly fewer years and opportunities to contribute to and engage in the development of nursing science to improve practice and care. "Ultimately, it is the health of the public that loses," she concluded.

Bleich said additional nurse scientists are needed to be part of the interdisciplinary research dialogue. Nurses bring a needed lens to research teams that gather, analyze, and look at new interventional models and understand the health care system and policy.

Tagliareni added that multiple entry points are needed to create more minority nurse researchers. When mentoring and funding are available, minority nurses can move from these multiple access points into advanced practice and research.

Future Directions for Advanced Education

Each discussant offered recommendations about advanced education of nurses for the committee's consideration.

Cronenwett said many of the funds for nursing education currently included in general medical education funding should be redirected to support either graduate nurse education or "transition to practice" residency programs. Additionally, she said policies should ensure that schools produce increasing numbers of nurse practitioners for primary care roles because expanded access to health care will increase society's need for primary care providers.

Tagliareni urged a reconfiguration, rethinking, and refocus on recognizing the value of nurse educators. Academic nursing education should be valued as a specialty area of practice and as an advanced practice role within the nursing profession. Tracks within master's and D.N.P. programs should focus on developing specialized knowledge, skills, and abilities that are specific to nurse educators.

Fulmer advocated teaching complex geriatric syndrome content and chronic care management in family- and patient-centered contexts. Few nursing educators who teach geriatrics are certified in the field, she said. She also urged that education about team and collaborative care be integrated into nursing curriculums in new ways.

Salmon said the importance of nursing science and its contributions to improving care and health should be raised on the national agenda. Greater support for predoctoral and postdoctoral nursing education, with an emphasis on training in research-intense environments, is needed. This would allow scientists to begin their careers earlier, with a stronger training trajectory, and would provide the benefit of working collaboratively with interdisciplinary colleagues.

QUESTION AND ANSWER SESSION

During the question and answer session with the committee, the armchair discussants focused largely on how nursing education should change as health care increasingly migrates from acute care settings into the community. Nurses must be able to work within the community and to shift care toward prevention to the greatest extent possible, said Salmon. Cronenwett said what people in a nursing home or in their own homes want is for nurses to apply to the community the skills and knowledge used in acute care settings. The notion of where nurses should work needs to be broadened, but "I am very reluctant not to produce the generic, generalist graduate who is capable of doing work in acute care and/or the community," Cronenwett concluded.

Fulmer pointed out that the infrastructure for community health care and education are not where they need to be. Nurses and interdisciplinary thinkers need to ask what will enable a new nursing graduate to practice more autonomously in a setting where they will not have colleagues readily available for collaboration and brainstorming.

The education of a nurse should be based on liberal learning and engagement in society at large, Salmon said. Nursing is part of the fabric of society, and nurses should be leaders in society.

3

How to Teach

Health care needs in the United States have changed over time, said Dr. Linda Burnes Bolton, vice president for nursing, chief nursing officer, and director of nursing research at Cedars-Sinai Medical Center. After World War II, many people returned from the war with specific health care needs, and the nursing education system at the time was inadequate to meet those needs. Today the aging of the U.S. population has created a new set of needs and new strains on nursing education. "How do we ensure the availability of a qualified workforce that is able to meet the public's needs?" Burnes Bolton asked. "That is part of our work on the Initiative on the Future of Nursing."

Burnes Bolton moderated the second armchair discussion, which examined the topic "How to Teach." This armchair discussion featured five education experts: Dr. Divina Grossman, founding vice president of engagement and former dean of Nursing & Health Sciences at Florida International University (FIU); Dr. Pamela R. Jeffries, associate dean of academic affairs at Johns Hopkins University School of Nursing; Cathleen Krsek, director of quality operations at the University Health-System Consortium (UHC); Dr. Robert W. Mendenhall, president of Western Governors University (WGU); and Dr. John A. Rock, senior vice president for medical affairs and founding dean of the Herbert Wertheim College of Medicine at FIU. Burnes Bolton asked the discussants to describe the strategies their respective institutions have adopted to improve the education of nurses. She also asked them to provide their recommendations to the committee for advancing the mechanisms used to educate students. The discussants focused on innovations in technology, online learning, nurse residency programs, and interprofessional collaborations that are being used across the country to improve access to high-quality educational opportunities for nurses at all levels.

TECHNOLOGY IN NURSING EDUCATION

One way to ensure the availability of a qualified workforce is through the enhanced use of technology, Jeffries said. Nursing education today is very "siloed." There are theory classes with lectures and Power-Point presentations and laboratories where students learn specific skills. "Then, by magic, we take [nurses] to a clinical practicum where they are supposed to be putting everything together and [demonstrating a] higher order of learning and critical thinking. But they have never practiced that," Jeffries asserted. The use of technology in nursing education offers opportunities to break down some of the silos and prepare students for decision making in complex care environments.

Learning Through Simulation

Simulations employing technology can allow students to practice skills, learn professional behavior, and demonstrate clinical reasoning in a safe environment, Jeffries said. Though more evidence is needed on the outcomes of using simulations as a teaching strategy, it engages students and provides them with higher-level learning opportunities they have not had before, such as clinical decision making, prioritization, and delegation skills.

Clinical simulations can be incorporated across theory, laboratory, and clinical courses. If done correctly, simulations enable a student-centered approach in which students are immersed in situations where they have to solve problems and think critically. "Every time I see students in simulations, I learn something new," Jeffries said. The most critical component of a simulation is the debriefing afterward; this process of guided reflection is where students learn the most. "They don't know what they don't know until you immerse them in a simulation," she said.

The use of simulations has exploded in the past 5 years, and federal funding may further increase their use. Regional "sim" centers are being built across the country and around the world, Jeffries said. More advanced simulators that replicate human responses are on the way. Virtual-world and second-life simulations will also be used more.

E-Learning and Mobile Devices

E-learning, which employs a variety of electronic media to promote learning, also offers great potential for nursing education, according to Jeffries. It provides students with the educational mobility to take courses and learn any time and anywhere. It also provides many students and practicing nurses with an opportunity to advance their careers—opportunities that may not have been available for some students if e-learning were not available.

Mobile devices are also valuable in nursing education. They include hand-held devices known as "clickers" for use in classes, personal digital assistants for use at the point of care, clinical information systems, and other technologies that are readily available and portable. Some of these devices are expensive, but "we have to teach students how to use these technological devices by incorporating them into the curriculum because they are used across clinical settings and teach students real-life skills," Jeffries said. The use of technology also engages students in active learning, such as when the clickers are used in a classroom to elicit student participation and responses during lectures.

A number of studies have compared traditional instructional methods with technology-based methods; many of these studies have found no significant differences (Jeffries et al., 2002, 2003). However, at other times, students learning through e-learning platforms and in online environments are more satisfied with the format and are learning just as much (Armstrong and Frueh, 2003; Billings and Halstead, 2009; Buckley, 2003; Simonson et al., 2000; Wills and Stommel, 2002). For example, outcomes data are appearing on the use of simulations to teach specific skills, such as pediatric resuscitation (Cheng et al., 2009; Childs and Sepples, 2006; Rauen, 2001). As simulations, e-learning, and mobile devices become more sophisticated, they will be merged so that learning can take place 24/7. Today's students embrace technology, which means that technology offers a tremendous opportunity to enhance teaching and learning, Jeffries said.

Advancing the Use of Technology in Education

The largest barrier to greater use of technologies is convincing faculty to use them, Jeffries noted. Faculty members may not know how to use technologies, or they may believe that students cannot learn content this way. But e-learning and the use of technology in education is here to stay, she said. Faculty development is needed in using this pedagogy and capturing data to measure outcomes.

Jeffries made two recommendations for the committee's consideration. First, educators must be willing to try new, innovative strategies to engage students. To create this willingness, faculty should be provided with development opportunities in the use of technologies. Like students, faculty members "don't know what they don't know" unless they learn about new devices and technologies and their potential. It is difficult for educators to embrace simulations if they are not informed and do not have experience in these areas. The Health Resources and Services Administration is providing funding in that area, and this funding should continue, said Jeffries.

Federal funding could also be used to identify standards and perform evaluations of simulations. With the current lack of standards, a simulation used in Ohio might be very different from one in Iowa. Additionally, the proportional use of simulations as a substitute for clinical experience varies from place to place, noted Jeffries.

ONLINE EDUCATION

The WGU online nursing program offers a variety of nursing programs, including a B.S.N. for initial licensure, R.N. to B.S.N., R.N. to M.S.N., and two master's degree programs. Launched in 2009, more than 600 nursing students are now enrolled from all 50 states. Tuition is $6,500 per 12-month year; the program is self-sustaining on tuition and requires no external support. Didactic instruction is delivered online while hospital partners provide clinical rotations, coaches, and clinical supervisors. WGU offers a B.S.N. for initial licensure in partnership with major hospitals, including Cedars-Sinai, Hospital Corporation of America, Kaiser Permanente, and Tenet. The success of the WGU program answers an important question in nursing education, Mendenhall said, "How do we create systems that are scalable, affordable, and have a greater throughput of students?"

Competency-Based Education

"What makes our nursing programs unique is that we are entirely competency-based," Mendenhall said. Competencies are defined by nursing practitioners using nursing standards. Using a student-centric model, students demonstrate competency by passing a series of assessments, including objective tests, performance tests, and clinical tests. "When they can demonstrate that they have mastered the competencies, they graduate," he said.

Adult learners come to higher education knowing different things and learning at different paces. Yet traditionally the education system has determined that everyone needs the same courses and the same number of credit hours and that every course should take 4 months. "We have tried to remove those barriers and teach students the way they learn—giving them self-paced, technology-based learning materials that they can do at their own pace," Mendenhall said. Students move quickly through what they know and take as much time as they need to learn materials they do not know, with content delivered through interactive, self-paced modules.

Faculty and Students

WGU hires faculty who are interested in the online education model and who went into nursing education because they wanted to work with students. New faculty participate in an extensive, month-long training and development program before they begin teaching and interacting with students. All new instructors are paired with an experienced faculty mentor for a year as they gradually increase the number of students they teach. Faculty members typically have 32 hours of contact time with students per week via telephone, e-mail, Web discussions, and threaded discussion groups. The role of faculty at WGU has changed from delivering content to being mentors of students; their full-time role is guiding, coaching, and directing students while answering questions and leading discussions.

Students, meanwhile, are part of online learning communities where they can collaborate with each other and with faculty. "Faculty stay with students from the day they start until the day they graduate, so we judge faculty based on the retention rates, graduation rates, student progress rates, and student satisfaction," Mendenhall said. The WGU program has a 50:1 faculty:student ratio as opposed to a more typical 10:1 ratio. Yet, Mendenhall noted, independent national surveys indicate that students report more interaction with their online faculty than do students in brick-and-mortar institutions.

The Use of Technology

Technology can also be used to improve clinical education, Mendenhall said. Most states require a specific number of hours of clinical experience. However, few define what must actually occur during that clinical time. The WGU online program has defined a set of clinical competencies and has used those competencies to develop simulations that teach students essential clinical skills. Experiences in clinical settings tend to be random—whatever happens on that day is what is experienced. On the other hand, scenarios can be planned using simulation so that experiences are consistent and every student has the same opportunities to master the same skills and competencies. Simulations are also more effective than clinical practice in allowing students to practice their skills repeatedly in a safe environment. "The clinical rotations are more effective if students are able to use what they have already mastered in simulations," Mendenhall said.

Expanding Capacity and Improving Education

During the armchair discussion, Mendenhall offered a number of recommendations for the committee's consideration in terms of improving the education of nurses, especially through the use of technology and online education.

Nursing education has severely constrained capacity, and tens of thousands of qualified applicants are turned away from nursing school every year. "We don't have the ability to expand that capacity unless we find new ways to teach. In my view, technology is the only real answer to significantly expanding our capacity for teaching in a cost-effective manner," Mendenhall said. Technology is required to leverage faculty time and clinical spaces to increase nursing education capacity. According to Mendenhall, simulation must become a greater percentage of clinical experiences—at least half—and regulatory requirements need to be changed to allow for this. "If we are not willing to use technology, and in particular simulations, we are not going to magically get twice as many clinical spots," he concluded.

Mendenhall also indicated that institutional and regulatory requirements need to be changed from hours to competencies, both for didactic and for clinical learning. "It's important to measure learning rather than time," he said.

NURSE RESIDENCY PROGRAMS

The first few years of practice can be difficult for new nurses. Turnover rates as high as 60 percent have been reported in the first year of nursing, and the most recent national data, collected in 2007 by PricewaterhouseCoopers' Health Research Institute, indicated a 27 percent turnover rate in the first year (PricewaterhouseCoopers' Health Research Institute, 2007). Nurse residency programs can reduce these difficulties, said Krsek.

Although many question the cost-effectiveness of nurse residency programs, these programs can generate considerable savings by reducing high rates of turnover. Cheryl Jones, associate professor at the University of North Carolina School of Nursing, has calculated that the expense for each new graduate who leaves nursing in the first year is $88,000 (Jones, 2008). By contrast, UHC has calculated that the expense for a residency program is approximately $50,000 to $75,000 for administration and approximately $900 to $1,000 per resident, which is ultimately much less than the turnover costs. "That is a tremendous return on investment," Krsek said. In fact, the Methodist Hospital System in Houston has estimated an 884 percent return on investment after its turnover rate fell from 50 percent to 13 percent in one year, with further reductions in subsequent years to less than 5 percent following the implementation of a residency program (Pine and Tart, 2007). Krsek said the UHC/American Association of Colleges of Nursing (AACN) Nurse Residency Program had a turnover rate of 4.4 percent last year.

Easing Transitions

Nurses enter the workforce as advanced beginners and need support as they transition to becoming competent professionals, Krsek said. They come out of school with a solid theoretical foundation, but they need to be able to apply that knowledge and develop their situational decision making. "It takes about a year for a new graduate to become competent, so they are left after orientation expecting to be able to fully function, yet they don't feel functional," Krsek explained.

Residency programs give nurses a way to learn to feel functional. Typical programs cover topics such as conflict management, interdisciplinary communication, diversity, and nurse-sensitive outcomes. During the program, nurses work with an advanced practice nurse in a nonthreatening arena away from clinical situations, said Krsek. All of the residents in the UHC/AACN program are also required to do an evidence-based project in the second half of their residency year.

The National Council of State Boards of Nursing recommends a residency program for newly licensed nurses (NCSBN, 2009). Additionally, Patricia Benner and her associates, in their new book, *Educating Nurses: A Call for Radical Transformation*, call for a 1-year residency program for all new graduates to support the clinical application of theoretical knowledge (Benner et al., 2009). Residency programs produce "safe, quality, competent care with a stable workforce," said Krsek.

Krsek had just one recommendation for the committee's consideration: Organizations should provide the resources to support the transition to practice of new graduates with 1-year residence programs. These residencies also could take place in community-based settings, she said.

A MODEL FOR INTERDISCIPLINARY EDUCATION

Florida International University, as described by Grossman and Rock, is a research university that serves a diverse student body. FIU has a new college of medicine and is in the early stages of implementing a community-centric, interprofessional program called Neighborhood HELP (Health Education Learning Program). This program will integrate classroom learning, community experiences, and clinical activities for students in medicine, nursing, social work, public health, and allied professions, including occupational therapy, physical therapy, speech/language pathology, and dietetics and nutrition.

Curricular and Pedagogical Goals

An interprofessional team of faculty has been meeting since fall 2008 to develop a community-based curriculum and pedagogical strategies for course content and clinical activities. As part of the curriculum, medical, nursing, and social work students will be required to take an interprofessional course that will cover topics such as quality and safety, crosscultural communication, collaboration, conflict management, professional bias, and leadership. The class will also include case-based group discussions and visits to community agencies and hospitals to observe interprofessional care teams in action.

The cornerstone of the Neighborhood HELP program is the community-based clinical experience and education. Interprofessional teams of students, including medical, nursing, and social work students, will be assigned to 2 of 1,400 households in underserved communities that have agreed to participate and were identified in collaboration with community leaders and stakeholders. The medical students will work with these two households for the 4-year duration of their academic programs and will partner with nursing students at different levels of education. For example, first-year medical students will be partnered with junior nursing students, while fourth-year students will be partnered with nurse practitioner students.

Students working with these households will be able to assess the health care and social service needs of families, learn about the social determinants of health, identify gaps in health care, provide health education, and make referrals to appropriate community agencies. Beginning in May 2010, the nursing, medical, and social work students will conduct regular household visits. During those visits, student teams will interview family members about their health, conduct standardized assessments of their social service and health needs, and collaboratively develop and implement a health care plan. Expected outcomes include improvements to quality of life and health in these neighborhoods, increased health literacy, and effective interprofessional communication and collaboration among faculty and students in the teams.

Links with the Community

FIU was fortunate in that it recently established a new medical school after the schools of nursing and public health were already in place and active, which meant that the medical school did not have a preestablished culture, Rock said. "We could think completely outside the box" in making the school patient- and community-centric and with a curriculum based in the community, he said. Over the past 2.5 years, FIU has been able to develop relationships with the primary cultural stakeholders represented in the community, including leaders in the Hispanic, African-American, Haitian, and Jewish communities. Additional community partners include neighborhood businesses, the fire department, the police department, the schools, faith-based organizations, primary care providers, and the Jackson Health System. "We have the entire loop covered," said Rock, "when we are in households, the patients can be redirected to a community health center, and if they are admitted into the hospital our students can go there and then return home with them."

The social mission of Neighborhood HELP program is "to improve the quality of life for the citizens of South Florida household by household," Rock said. At the same time, the program will be able to train "culturally competent students who celebrate diversity and appreciate the wonderful benefits from understanding different cultures and the challenges they have in meeting a variety of health care needs."

Traditionally, Rock said, outcomes were measured by the numbers of graduates successfully matriculated by a program. But another important part of an institution's mission should be to improve the quality of life of a neighborhood or community. "That is another return of investment on the educational dollar. We have this huge amount of good will among our students who want to do good when they come to be educated. We have not effectively used that energy to meet the challenges we have in our neighborhoods," he concluded.

Improving Education Through Collaboration

Grossman and Rock had several recommendations for the committee to consider with regard to improving education through interprofessional collaboration and community partnerships:

- Use a community-centric approach in education so that students learn through discovery how to improve health not only for individuals, but also for families and communities;
- Create more interprofessional education models to socialize students to teamwork and cooperative learning;

- Provide leadership from the top by having deans of nursing, medicine, public health, and social work model interprofessional collaboration; and
- Transcend issues of turf, tradition, and power so that interprofessional education models can flourish.

QUESTION AND ANSWER SESSION

During the question and answer session, one committee member asked Rock about the best ways to establish interprofessional collaboration and partnerships between nursing and medical schools in situations where the medical school is already well established. Rock said that collaboration has to be endorsed by the institution or university as a whole and become a mandated challenge. Interprofessional collaboration needs to become part of a consensus among stakeholders and be incorporated into a redefined strategic program. Another member of the committee asked about the cost of the model at FIU compared to a more conventional classroom approach to health professional education. Rock answered that the pedagogy is embedded in the curriculum, so it is part of the overall cost of the medical school and is treated as a fixed cost. Grossman noted that the establishment of the program is part of a curriculum redesign that integrates all aspects of the program, effectively shifting the costs. Additionally, FIU has received funding from several foundations to endow the program in perpetuity, in part because of the benefits to the community of having such a program.

In response to a question about how to achieve interdisciplinary collaboration through an online community, Mendenhall said that capturing the interdisciplinary nature of education remains an evolving challenge in online education, especially because WGU does not have a medical school or other institutions at which students may work. Instead, WGU partners with acute care centers and community health centers to provide students with practical experiences and expose them to other professions in the clinical setting. Mendenhall explained that at WGU, the clinical experience for students is based on cohorts. Students are organized into groups that become part of online learning communities that interact with each other. Mendenhall also said that the WGU program defines the competencies that are needed, including interdisciplinary competencies, and finds the best content available, regardless of the source.

4

Where to Teach

The topic "Where to Teach" in nursing education inevitably overlaps with the previous armchair discussions that explored the topics "What to Teach" and "How to Teach," said Jennie Chin Hansen, senior fellow at the Center for the Health Professions of the University of California–San Francisco, and 2008–2010 president of AARP, who moderated the third armchair discussion at the forum. Schools and educational programs operate in dynamic environments with a variety of factors that define and shape the education of nurses and health care providers across the nation. Few medical or nursing schools can be created from the ground up, meaning that institutions inevitably need to deal with existing structures—both physical and administrative—and cultures. At the same time, job demands, institutional resources, and available technologies are constantly changing and influencing the direction of nursing education. Meanwhile, cities and states need to plan for their own futures and identify the health needs of their populations, which means that educational and health care institutions become economic and civic concerns.

Led by Chin Hansen, this armchair discussion included insights from four experts in nursing education: Dr. Willis N. Holcombe, chancellor of the Florida College System; Catherine Rick, chief nursing officer for the Department of Veterans Affairs; Dr. Christine A. Tanner, A. B. Youmans-Spaulding Distinguished Professor for the School of Nursing at the Oregon Health & Science University (OHSU); and Rose Yuhos, executive director of the Area Health Education Center of Southern Nevada. The armchair discussion examined several unique, successful models of nursing education that have transcended traditional classroom models of education. Discussants also identified a number of unresolved questions. As Chin Hansen said, quoting a speaker from the first forum on the future of nursing that focused on acute care, "the future is here, it's just not everywhere."

THE EDUCATION CONSORTIUM MODEL

One of the most pressing challenges facing the nursing profession is how to prepare nurses who can be responsive to emerging health care needs and practice in the rapidly changing health care environment, given that the capacity of the education system is limited by faculty shortages and lack of clinical training sites, Tanner said. The state of Oregon has taken an innovative approach to nursing education by not focusing exclusively on the degrees that nurses should earn, Tanner noted. Instead, the state has framed its improvement efforts in nursing education around the competencies that nurses need to practice effectively and the capacity required to educate these nurses. To achieve these overlapping goals, the Oregon Consortium for Nursing Education (OCNE) was established in 2001. The consortium consists of eight community colleges and five campuses of OHSU.

The Consortium Curriculum

To establish a common education base, the consortium faculty created a shared nursing curriculum that is used on all participating community college and OHSU campuses. The curriculum redefines the fundamentals of nursing to reflect health promotion, evidence-based practice, clinical judgment, relationship-centered care, and leadership. The competencies that are integrated into the curriculum were identified based on an analysis of emerging health care needs and alternative scenarios of how the practice of nursing could change to address those needs. For example, the curriculum includes two courses in the management of chronic illnesses, reflecting the changing demographics of Americans and the need to help students gain competencies in those areas. The curriculum also has an integrative practicum that was developed to provide a better transition to practice for nursing students.

When accepted into the OCNE program, students are co-admitted into both the associate and baccalaureate degree programs. This provides a seamless transition for students who start the program in a community college and move into the baccalaureate program at the university. "We are trying to eliminate every barrier to students continuing for a bachelor's degree," said Tanner. The curriculum is viewed as a continuous course of study that students can complete in 4 years.

In addition to the shared curriculum and co-admission, the OCNE program features shared instructional resources, faculty who teach across campuses to maximize use of available expertise, and continued innovation in classroom and clinical instruction, said Tanner. The consortium is committed to incorporating best practices into teaching and learning throughout the curriculum. It is creating a new clinical education model that integrates simulation throughout the education of nurses. "We are rolling that [model] out on four of our campuses and evaluating the outcomes," Tanner noted.

Advancing Community College and University Partnerships

Tanner offered three recommendations for the committee's consideration:

- Create new nursing education systems that use existing resources in community colleges and universities and provide for common prerequisites, a competency-based nursing curriculum, and shared instructional resources;
- Convene one or more expert panels to develop a model prelicensure curriculum that can be used as a framework by faculty in community college–university partnerships. This model prelicensure curriculum should be used as the basis for local curriculum, be based on emerging health care needs, incorporate widely accepted nursing competencies, as interpreted for new care delivery models, and integrate best practices in teaching and learning; and
- Invest in a national initiative to develop and evaluate new approaches to prelicensure clinical education, including a required postgraduate residency under a restricted license.

BACCALAUREATES THROUGH
COMMUNITY COLLEGES

The state of Florida has identified three workforce shortage areas where it is not producing enough graduates to meet growing demands within the state: teaching, nursing, and applied technology, Holcombe said. In 2009, the Florida legislature questioned why the Florida College System[1] could not help close workforce gaps by going beyond associate degrees to produce graduates with baccalaureate degrees in the defined shortage areas. The system, which is made up of 28 community colleges, has responded to this challenge. So far, 14 of the 28 community colleges in the Florida College System have been given the authority to grant baccalaureate degrees, 9 of which are now granting baccalaureate degrees in nursing (B.S.N.s).

Relationships Among Institutions

Establishing baccalaureate degree programs within the community college system required significant collaboration among institutions within the public university system, Holcombe noted. Universities and private colleges in the state have an opportunity to weigh in on proposals made by the community colleges in generating new baccalaureate degree programs. As new programs are instituted, the feedback process has provided collaboration beyond the faculty level to the overall higher education system in Florida. "If there is not collaboration and dialogue, the program does not go forward and does not get approval," he said.

Florida must continue to build on its associate degrees in nursing (A.D.N.) programs as a base because of the state's acute nursing shortage, Holcombe stated. If new competencies must be mastered by nurses, then the curriculums of the A.D.N. programs must be revised to incorporate these new expectations. More than two-thirds of nurses in Florida come through associate degree programs, so the colleges are expanding these programs even as they begin establishing their baccalaureate degree programs.

---

[1]The Florida College System was previously known as the Florida Community College System.

Advancing the Education Pipeline

During his remarks, Holcombe offered two recommendations to the committee in terms of advancing education and advancing nurses within the education pipeline to achieve higher levels of competence and education:

- Include associate degree nursing programs in the dialogue about "What to Teach" so that new competencies are incorporated into all nursing education programs; and
- Increase the emphasis on creating opportunities for educational advancement from A.D.N. to B.S.N. to M.S.N. and beyond. These opportunities should be widely available, collaborative among institutions including both community colleges and universities, and technologically sophisticated.

ACADEMIC-PRACTICE PARTNERSHIPS

The Veterans Health Administration under the Department of Veterans Affairs (VA) has four key missions: providing clinical care, educating and preparing health professionals, researching across the continuum of scientific endeavors, and providing backup for the Department of Defense in areas such as emergency preparedness. All four of those goals require having great talent in the VA system, said Rick.

Developing Human Capital

The integrated VA health care system provides a full range of services across the care continuum, including acute, primary, home health, and long-term care and telehealth services. The system has more than 75,000 nursing personnel, including more than 55,000 Registered Nurses (R.N.s). These nurses fill vital roles, including leadership positions, staff clinicians, clinical nurse leaders, nurse informaticians, clinical nurse specialists, and nurse practitioners. Approximately 22,000 of these R.N.s are eligible for retirement in 2010, Rick said.

To identify and meet its human capital needs, the VA Office of Nursing Services developed a national nursing strategic plan in 2000 that emphasized career development and workforce management. In 2002, a

2-year external commission on the future of nursing at the VA, chaired by Linda Burnes Bolton, recommended that the VA establish a nursing academic model similar to its medical academic model. A model of this type would promote VA partnerships with the academic community to leverage available resources, increase research within VA practice settings, and realize the potential for enhanced recruitment and retention. In 2005, the VA began an early initiative to respond to the commission's recommendation to develop academic-practice partnerships and recognize the need for faculty development. The program was called TEACH (Transforming Educational Affiliations for Clinical Horizons). It offered small block grants to VA health care facilities to create innovative partnerships with academic affiliates.

The VA Nursing Academy

Building on the TEACH program and the promise of academic-practice partnerships, the VA launched the VA Nursing Academy (VANA) in 2007. VANA is a 5-year, $40 million pilot program. Its primary goals are to develop partnerships with academic nursing institutes, expand the number of faculty for baccalaureate programs, establish partnerships to enhance faculty development, and increase baccalaureate enrollment to increase the nursing supply, not solely for the VA, but for the country at large. It also was aimed at encouraging interprofessional programs and increasing the retention and recruitment of VA nurses.

The program has been in place for 2.5 years; in that time, three cycles of requests for proposals were sent to more than 600 colleges and schools of nursing, as well as to institutions within the VA system. Fifteen geographically and demographically diverse pilot sites were selected to participate in VANA based on the strength of their proposals, Rick noted. The third cycle of requests also emphasized creating a cohort of smaller facilities because they were not competing in the program as well as the highly academic, urban universities and institutions.

Measuring Outcomes

Each funded VANA partnership is required to have a rigorous evaluation plan to measure outcomes, Rick explained. Outcomes observed by the partnerships are expected to include increased staff, patient, student, and faculty satisfaction; greater scholarly output; enhanced professional development; better continuity and coordination of care; more reliance on evidence-based practice; and enhanced interprofessional learning. Each selected school is also expected to increase enrollment by at least 20 students a year.

The initial evidence regarding faculty recruitment and retention has been "very positive," Rick said. She highlighted a number of innovative strategies that have been implemented across VANA partnerships. Faculty have been embedded within designated educational units, commonly referred to as DEUs, to work on evidence-based practice projects. Advanced residency and internship programs have been developed and implemented, and institutions have developed clinical nurse leader programs. Adjunct VA faculty have been added as guest lecturers, instructors, and researchers, and students have been given new clinical opportunities.

Altogether the program has resulted in 2,700 new students, with 620 receiving the majority of their clinical rotation experiences at the VA, Rick said. The number of nursing school faculty has increased by 176, and the number of VA faculty by 264.

Advancing Academic-Practice Partnerships

In her concluding remarks, Rick offered the committee recommendations for advancing nursing education. Educational programs must prepare nurses for varied levels of complex roles, with degree-granting strategies designed to address defined competencies and parity with partners in health care teams, said Rick. Growing evidence points to improvements in efficiency and effectiveness related to nursing practice that supports master's-prepared nurse clinicians at the point of care and doctoral preparation for advanced practice roles.

Academic-practice partnerships that increase the numbers of clinicians who teach and the number of faculty who practice are essential to meeting the educational needs of nursing. This may require restructuring of accreditation standards or legislated incentives, Rick said. Such partnerships should include internships and residencies that provide appropriate clinical experiences, with defined structures for instruction that align practice and academic approaches for all levels of nursing in wide-ranging roles and settings.

AREA HEALTH EDUCATION CENTERS

Area Health Education Centers (AHECs) link communities with academic and nursing practice by developing clinical rotation experiences for students, said Yuhos of Southern Nevada's AHEC. These centers are distributed throughout the nation and have traditionally been funded and operated through medical schools. However, in states without medical schools, health science institutions are beginning to apply for and develop AHEC programs. The centers have developed their clinical practice model around a medical education model, but are moving toward a clinical practice model that is more community focused. This shift and additional involvement from other disciplines, such as nursing, have fostered a move toward interdisciplinary training experiences for a broad array of health science students.

Yuhos described an AHEC system in Nevada that had created an interdisciplinary training experience in which teams of students participate in case-based learning that focuses on providing patient-centered care. This AHEC is in a rural ambulatory clinical setting that provides students with an opportunity to work in a resource-scarce environment. Teams are encouraged to use innovative techniques that stretch the boundaries of the team to include the community, Yuhos explained.

Developing Teamwork

In the AHEC training environment, students have an opportunity to represent their discipline while participating as active members and leaders of teams. For many students, these are new and different experiences. For example, in some cases nursing students are given an opportunity to lead a team, while medical students play more of a supporting role. These opportunities help students learn about the dynamics of working in interdisciplinary teams and provide them with competencies in leadership and team support, which are not traditionally taught. Participating in a collaborative team also allows students "to appreciate the diversity of what each discipline brings to the team and to the concept of care for that patient or that community," Yuhos said.

At the same time, faculty who participate in the AHEC model become more clinically experienced and benefit from providing students with training experiences in interdisciplinary teams. The AHEC model creates an environment where faculty need to work across disciplines to design unique experiences and programs that feature their own discipline as well as others.

Use of Simulations

In the future, clinical simulations will play an important role in the development of skill-based training for students, Yuhos said. "But I firmly believe that it is, and always will be, important to get the student in the community, so he or she can experience community dynamics that they can't experience in the sim lab," she said. Future nursing education in the future will occur in both the sim lab and the community. Students should be in the community, working with families and learning about the socioeconomic, cultural, and ethnic dynamics of families. The community has to be an important part of each student's experience, Yuhos concluded.

Advancing Interdisciplinary Collaboration

Yuhos had two recommendations for the committee to consider in regard to enhancing nursing education through the use of interdisciplinary collaboration:

- Identify and promote evidence-based clinical training models that include nursing students as part of the interdisciplinary team; and
- Identify and promote evidence-based interdisciplinary faculty development and clinical training models that include nurses as part of the interdisciplinary team.

QUESTION AND ANSWER SESSION

During a brief question and answer session with the committee, the discussants focused on advancing interprofessional education. Tanner and Rick concurred that interprofessional education is a valuable aspect of nursing education. Tanner said that successful interprofessional education requires a strategic initiative that has both grassroots support and support from university leadership and administration. She noted that a great deal of grassroots work has been done with regional Oregon AHECs to establish interprofessional clinical experiences for health professional students in rural settings. It is very important that students across the state have an opportunity to work collaboratively, no matter where the setting is located.

Rick noted that the VANA program includes interprofessional collaboration as part of its scoring criteria for selection of its partners. She noted that bridges need to be built to overcome some of the challenges and culture differences that have been experienced between the practice and academic communities, as well as across the different disciplines. Rick described one of the promising models that had been featured as part of a possible pilot; the model included nurses as formal preceptors for medical students. She said interprofessional collaboration is ingrained in the vision of the VANA program, and perhaps one day the nursing academy could instead be called the interprofessional academy.

5

Testimony

Prior to the forum in Houston, a variety of stakeholders and the public were invited to submit written testimony to the committee in three areas relevant to nursing education: what to teach, how to teach, and where to teach. Those submitting written testimony were asked to describe innovative models in these three areas: funding strategies and financial incentives that could be used in nursing education; barriers to implementing or expanding innovative models and programs being used in nursing education; and how nursing education could be improved to better meet the current and future needs of Americans. Those submitting testimony were also asked to share their overall vision of the future of nursing.

Twelve individuals at the forum provided prepared oral testimony for the Initiative on the Future of Nursing; in most cases, these individuals or the organizations they represented had also submitted written testimony for the committee's consideration. Many important ideas and suggestions for the initiative emerged from this testimony and are summarized below. A number of other individuals attending the forum offered ad hoc observations and opinions on what was discussed at the forum during an open-microphone session that closed the forum. These comments are summarized at the end of this chapter. Like the comments made by the discussants during the armchair discussions, the testimony, observations, and opinions in this chapter should not be interpreted as positions or recommendations of the committee, the Robert Wood Johnson Foundation (RWJF), or the Institute of Medicine (IOM). The testimony and comments made at the forum only represent the perspectives of those who attended and spoke at the forum and are not inclusive of all facets of nursing education.

James Walker, President
American Association of Nurse Anesthetists

Nurses need to develop an evidence-based perspective during their education to improve health care, control its costs, and extend patient access to care, said James Walker, president of the 40,000-member American Association of Nurse Anesthetists and director of Nursing Anesthesia for Baylor College of Medicine.

To become a certified registered nurse anesthetist (C.R.N.A.), a nurse must earn a bachelor's degree, become a licensed registered nurse, and practice in acute care for at least 1 year. Today, C.R.N.A.s are prepared at the master's level and take classes in pharmacology, anatomy, physiology, pathophysiology, and principles of anesthesia practice; they also gain extensive clinical experience. Nurse anesthetist graduates must pass a comprehensive certification exam to become a C.R.N.A., with recertification required every 2 years. By 2025, C.R.N.A.s will graduate from doctoral programs. Curricular content to be added in the future will focus on advancing clinical practice and research and improving the systems that shape anesthesia practice and care.

The outcome of the current educational system for nurse anesthetists is four-fold, Walker said:

1. It produces skilled nurse anesthetists to provide the full range of anesthesia and interventional pain management services.
2. It ensures patient access to care.
3. It creates access to surgical, trauma, interventional, diagnostic, and labor and delivery services everywhere in the country, particularly in rural and underserved areas of America.
4. It contributes to improving the quality of anesthesia care, which, according to the IOM, is approximately 50 times safer today than it was 20 years ago (IOM, 2000). This nurse-provided care is also a fraction of the cost associated with anesthesia provided by physician counterparts.

Given these outcomes, "there is now no place for restrictive federal barriers to nursing education practice," Walker said. "What the patients in our country need is for nurses to continue leading the way by example."

Diane Sosne, President
Service Employee International Union (SEIU) Healthcare 1199NW

To prepare nurses for leadership roles in tomorrow's health care system and to educate enough nurses to meet the nation's health care needs, nursing education must change, said Diane Sosne, president of SEIU Healthcare 1199NW in Washington state. Nursing education must emphasize safety, chronic disease management, preventive care, care coordination, the use of new technology, and multidisciplinary care delivery for diverse populations in multiple settings, including nontraditional ones. Providing such an education to nurses will create an important opportunity to increase the number and diversity of people in the nursing pipeline. "We need a tremendous number of nurses in all roles," Sosne said. Partnerships between labor and management can inform the design of programs and curriculums and build in support systems to help prospective nurses succeed.

Moving health care workers along a nursing career ladder enables them to build on prior learning and engage in continuous learning. Articulation between programs and the development of shared curriculums that connect various nursing programs and levels of education can provide financial efficiencies in education, Sosne said. It is very effective, for instance, to introduce nursing concepts in prerequisite courses and to contextualize these concepts in health care settings.

Sosne cited an example of a labor–management partnership in Seattle that involves SEIU Healthcare, Northwest Hospital, and North Seattle Community College. A biology prerequisite class is being supplemented with a simulation that integrates nursing processes and critical thinking into the class. Such innovations can be supported through public–private partnerships and can be "very successful," Sosne said, in leveraging the dollars invested in prerequisite and nursing education classes.

Phyllis Kritek, Conflict Engagement Consultant Trainer and Coach

Nursing education should build competencies in conflict engagement, said Phyllis Kritek, an independent conflict engagement consultant, trainer, and coach. Extensive research on patient safety has documented that the health care community has a cultural practice of avoiding, denying, and suppressing conflict, a practice that is often exacerbated by the abuse of power, she said. "Conflict competency is essential to challenge and change this culture," she added.

Professional nursing has a strong and proud tradition of advocating collaboration. The IOM reports *To Err Is Human* (2000) and *Keeping Patients Safe* (2004) were part of a process that helped demonstrate that the failure to collaborate is a key factor in adverse events and catalyzed the patient safety movement. Furthermore, conflict competency shifted from being an aspiration to a requirement when the Joint Commission specifically included wording on disruptive behaviors and conflict resolution in its 2009 Leadership Standards (Joint Commission, 2008).

All nursing curriculums should include conflict competency training, Kritek asserted. This training should move beyond oversimplifications and formulaic superficiality and emphasize relationship-based conflict engagement, which is the only approach that can ensure collaboration in the challenging situations nurses confront. "Our students need practical skills, not platitudes," she concluded.

Betty Young, President
Coleman College for Health Sciences, Houston Community College

Sergio Valdez was homeless in 2006 when he became an A.D.N. student at the Houston Community College Coleman College for Health Sciences. Today he is a registered nurse working at the Texas Medical Center. "This is just one person's story," said Betty Young, president of the Coleman College for Health Sciences at Houston Community College. "However, it is repeated day after day across the country in all of our community colleges." Students in community colleges earn not just their degrees, but also the confidence that they will be able to continue their education and be successful, contributing members of the community.

The average age of students at Coleman College is 32, which means that the average student has many things to think about that 18-, 19-, or

20-year-old students probably do not, Young said. Older students and their families may have to make many sacrifices to attend college. If these students are not given the chance to attend 2-year community college nursing programs and enter into practice, they may never attend college at all.

Young recommended that the A.D.N. program be maintained as the entry point for practice. "This contributes to the diverse population of nurse practice," Young said. Also, nurses should have an opportunity for continuing education, including earning a bachelor's degree, while also meeting the needs of their current employer and their personal goals, she concluded.

George Boggs, President and Chief Executive Officer (CEO)
American Association of Community Colleges (AACC)

Community colleges are the primary educators of the nation's new registered nurses, including the majority of underrepresented and returning nursing students, said AACC President and CEO George Boggs. A growing number of community colleges are offering B.S.N. programs, but the majority of nursing programs are taught at the associate degree level. The AACC favors more partnerships with university programs that are fully articulated, designed to facilitate life-long learning, and facilitate further education of associate degree nurses to help them earn advanced degrees and certifications. Especially important, said Boggs, are the R.N. to M.S.N. degree programs that can ease the persistent faculty shortages currently constraining nursing education.

Policies and regulations that encourage advanced degrees should not have the punitive effect of removing nurses from the workforce through the loss of their licenses, Boggs said. Options should be affordable; should recognize and give credit for education and experiences that nurses already have; and should be accessible even in remote and rural areas, where more than two-thirds of nurses are prepared in A.D.N. programs.

One option to consider is a 3-year B.S.N. program that is offered in other countries, Boggs said. This alternative to traditional 4-year programs could significantly increase the number of new B.S.N.s using the same available faculty and clinical site resources. Accreditation organizations may be reluctant to make such a dramatic change, but shared examinations could protect quality. "I urge the committee to focus on the quality of the outcome of the programs rather than recommending a limitation on how nurses are taught to one standard program type," Boggs said.

Cathleen Shultz, President
National League for Nursing (NLN)

Four values characterize the NLN's vision for the future of nursing—caring, integrity, diversity, and excellence—said NLN President Cathleen Shultz. She highlighted a number of specific areas where the nursing workforce will need additional expertise to meet the future needs of the population.

In the area of diversity, nursing education must establish a workforce of faculty, researchers, and scholars that moves beyond tolerance of differences to engagement and celebration of differences. "We must institutionalize a commitment to diversity," Shultz said. "Safe, quality care cannot be achieved without education inclusive of all."

The need is urgent to build a science of nursing and to prepare a technologically savvy workforce. Toward that goal, the NLN has created an innovative simulation and resource center that helps educators develop expertise in education methodologies specific to simulation. Additionally, with an aging population, nursing faculty must gain expertise in gerontology. Faculty development programs in geriatrics must be funded and gerontology must be integrated into the nursing curriculum, she said.

These complex areas make it abundantly clear that nursing education is an advanced specialty in its own right. The Academic Nurse Educator Certification Program has certified more than 2,000 certified nurse educators since its inception. This certification validates the knowledge educators need to practice the science of nursing education, Shultz explained.

Workforce issues are not going to go away soon, Shultz said. Nursing education must sidestep the argument over whether all nurses need bachelor's degrees and embrace the diversity offered by having multiple points of entry. All nurses should be encouraged and enabled to continue their education, she said. Problems in the work environment, such as inadequate compensation for nursing faculty, need to be confronted and creative solutions should be explored to recruit and retain faculty, Shultz concluded.

Tomika Harris
National Association of Pediatric Nurse Practitioners

As the nursing community looks to the future, it needs to consider three major issues, according to Tomika Harris, a faculty member at the University of Texas representing the National Association of Pediatric Nurse Practitioners.

First, the traditional nursing curriculum needs to be refocused to address the IOM's recommendation for shared health care competencies, such as patient-centered care, interdisciplinary teamwork, evidence-based practice, quality improvements, and informatics (IOM, 2003). Furthermore, it is imperative to evaluate shared competencies in terms of measurable outcomes, Harris said. "Nurses need to be prepared with the skills and competencies to provide safe, quality care," she said.

Second, nursing students at all levels need to have opportunities to integrate evidence-based research into their coursework and to engage in comparative effectiveness research that evaluates strategies to improve health, said Harris. The outcomes of this research provide essential information for clinicians and patients to decide on the best treatment. This research also provides criteria to improve the health of communities and to improve the health care system.

Third, nursing educators need to partner with funding organizations to provide seamless educational trajectories for all nursing specialties aimed at specific populations, said Harris. For example, geriatric nurses have successfully established a model partnership with the Hartford Foundation to support geriatric fellowships and innovative academic initiatives to revitalize interest in caring for the nation's elderly population in new and effective ways. Similar partnerships could encourage the establishment of consortiums of nursing schools, shared resources, and expertise aimed at developing shared skills and competencies in other areas, such as pediatrics, Harris said.

Alexia Green, Professor
Texas Tech University Health Sciences Center

Texas is the fastest growing state in the nation, adding nearly half a million new residents in 2009, surpassing California by nearly 100,000 new residents (U.S. Census Bureau, 2009), said Alexia Green, professor at the Texas Tech University Health Sciences Center and co-team leader of the Texas Team Addressing Nursing Education Capacity. Texas is also among the states with the largest uninsured and under-insured populations (Cunningham, 2010; Kaiser Family Foundation, *statehealthfacts.org*, 2010). To counter these tensions, the Texas Team developed a strategic plan that is supported by schools of nursing throughout the state, Green said.

The first goal is to focus on strategic growth and accountability, Green explained. Goals for enrollment growth in nursing education across the state have been set. Across the country, thousands of nurses are turned away from nursing programs, while thousands more enter nursing schools, but never graduate. "We need to address the [issue of] accountability," she said, "and we are attempting to do that within our state by making sure those nurses are successful."

The second goal is to establish regional collaboration among nursing schools across the state. Regional problems need to be identified and ad-dressed in a collaborative manner, said Green. For example, one area of focus is clinical simulations to meet the learning needs of students in ef-fective and efficient ways.

Mary Anne Dumas, President
National Organization of Nurse Practitioner Faculties

Educators of nurse practitioners (N.P.s) are highly innovative and adapt to working with limited resources to meet the needs of today's N.P. students, said Mary Anne Dumas, president of the National Organization of Nurse Practitioner Faculties. For example, as a result of the nursing faculty shortage and an increased faculty workload, N.P. educators are using technology to provide Web-based and distance learning to students and to other N.P. faculty. They are delivering curriculums to rural and international students 24 hours a day, 7 days a week. "Many students cannot go to school full-time and have to work to support their families and educational costs," Dumas said, and they "rely heavily on the flexi-bility of technology."

To accommodate different student learning styles and needs, faculty are using podcasts and streaming video to record lectures and entire courses, so that students can download and listen to or view them at any time. Blogs and Web-based discussions groups balance the convenience of technology with the interpersonal components of N.P. education, Dumas said.

Simulation labs are a "great learning tool" that enable students to develop skill sets that they may not experience in a clinical rotation, but simulations do not replace direct clinical experiences, Dumas said. However, making clinical sites available for student to achieve competence is a significant challenge for N.P. programs. "Competition for preceptors is fierce in areas with multiple programs," Dumas observed.

The challenge of access to clinical education sites could be reduced through dedicated funding for N.P. education that comes through academic institutions or community-based practice sites, Dumas said. Funding initiatives could provide reimbursement for N.P. education and increased support for nurse-managed health care centers, which are "ideal sites for exposing N.P. students to working with underserved populations," according to Dumas. Increased funds also could support the development of guidelines for practice, mentoring, leadership development, and other valuable experiences.

Fay Raines, President
American Association of Colleges of Nursing (AACN)

Education has a direct impact on the quality of care provided by nurses and on patient outcomes, said AACN President Fay Raines. "A more highly educated nursing workforce is essential for reforming health care, addressing quality failures, and meeting needs for primary care, geriatric care, and chronic care," she said.

Multiple studies demonstrate that outcomes improve when care is provided by nurses prepared at the baccalaureate level, and many national organizations, such as the Carnegie Foundation for the Advancement of Teaching, the National Advisory Council on Nurse Education and Practice, and the American Organization of Nurse Executives, have called for increasing the number of B.S.N.-prepared nurses. Raines also urged the committee to make recommendations for a more highly educated nursing workforce, which could be achieved by raising the educational level of nurses and reenvisioning traditional roles. As one step toward this goal, AACN is working with practice colleagues to implement the Clinical Nurse Leader Initiative. Partners in this effort include health care organizations, the Department of Veterans Affairs, and the nursing services of the Armed Forces.

The ability to prepare a well-educated nursing workforce depends on having large numbers of doctorally prepared nurses as educators, scientists, and expert clinicians. A stronger focus is needed on producing more entry-level nurses at the baccalaureate level, Raines said, because data show that nurses entering the profession with a bachelor's degree are almost four times more likely to pursue graduate studies (HRSA, 2006).

The education of advanced practice nurses also must be transformed. The growing number of nurses with doctorates of nursing practice (D.N.P.s) and recognition of the D.N.P. as the preferred preparation for specialty roles is a step in this direction, said Raines. More advanced practice nurses will be essential to meet the nation's primary health care needs. "If we are to safely care for patients and effectively prepare future clinicians, we must make raising the educational level of nurses a national priority," she concluded.

Patricia Hinton Walker, Vice President for Nursing Policy and
Professor of Nursing Uniformed Services
University of the Health Sciences

Discussions of the future of nursing need to focus on where technology will take health care in the future, not where technology is today, said Patricia Hinton Walker, vice president for nursing policy and professor of nursing at the Uniformed Services University of the Health Sciences. Speaking as chair of the Technology Informatics Guiding Education Reform (TIGER) Initiative, Hinton Walker noted that innovative technologies from companies such as Microsoft and CVS are already moving patients forward in a socially disruptive way. "We need to talk not only about the community as a partner, but patients as partners in a very different way," said Hinton Walker. She noted that the president of the National Committee for Quality Assurance recently referred to the "activated patient." In this respect, nursing education needs to view patients not as the objects of care, but as partners in practice.

The increased use of technologies, such as electronic health records, will have a profound effect on practice, education, and policy, said Hinton Walker. For example, electronic health records will play a vital role in comparative effectiveness research, which will "change how we define evidence in the future." Evidence-based medicine will still be based on randomized controlled trials, she said, but it will also be based on broader measures of the effects of the health care delivery system. To take another example, regional health information centers will influence nursing curriculums, assessments of education, the integration of ethics and policy into teaching, and the approaches taken to personalizing medicine. Data will be "the new knowledge of the future," Hinton Walker said.

The new capabilities that will be created by technology have not been a prominent part of the ongoing dialogue about nursing or interdisciplinary interactions in health care, Hinton Walker said. The TIGER Initiative urges the committee to consider how nurses need to be prepared for a technologically evolving future, she concluded.

David Longanecker, President
Western Interstate Commission for Higher Education

Retaining the associate's degree in nursing is crucial, said David Longanecker, president of the Western Interstate Commission for Higher Education (WICHE). "It is possible that the bachelor's degree for all entering nurses would be the perfect solution. But this is the best example I have seen in a long time where the perfect would be the enemy of the good," Longanecker pointed out.

The A.D.N. should not be eliminated for three reasons, Longanecker said. First, requiring a bachelor's degree for entry into practice is not affordable. For the 2007–2008 cohort of A.D.N. recipients, WICHE estimates that the cost of continuing on to a bachelor's degree would be $800 million in tuition, along with other costs of attending college, and would cost the states an additional $600 million in appropriations to take those students through an additional 2 years. "Neither the students nor the states can afford that," said Longanecker.

Second, retention of the A.D.N. is essential to diversify the nursing workforce. In Colorado, 20 percent of the population is Hispanic (U.S. Census Bureau, 2010), and that percentage will grow to 33 percent by 2025, according to estimates from the National Center for Higher Education Management Systems. However, just 3 percent of the nursing workforce is Hispanic, said Longanecker (HRSA, 2009). According to data from the National Center for Education Statistics, students of color have a greater representation in community colleges than in 4-year institutions—in 2008, 42 percent of community college students were from communities of color, compared with 32 percent of students at 4-year institutions, "and it appears likely that this will become even more skewed in years to come," Longanecker predicted.

Third, the resources are not available to increase the capacity of bachelor's programs in nursing. Especially in rural areas, the A.D.N. is crucial, and calculations by WICHE reveal that 20 percent of all A.D.N.s are conferred by rural institutions, compared with just 4 percent of bachelor's degrees in nursing, Longanecker noted.

More B.S.N.s are absolutely necessary, and the capacity of 4-year institutions should be increased to expand the number of nurses with bachelor's degrees. However, nursing also needs much stronger articulation programs and consortiums like the one in Oregon, said Longanecker. These programs provide professional tracks for more nurses to enter the field and then advance in the profession through work and learning.

CONCLUDING REMARKS

At the end of the forum, Donna E. Shalala, committee chair, invited members of the audience to share their concluding remarks with the committee. Many people offered their perspectives and insight on ideas that were heard during the event or anecdotal experiences in nursing education. This final open-microphone session yielded many observations from the audience on a variety of topics relevant to the committee's work and the future of nursing education. Like the testimony summarized above, these comments should not be interpreted as positions or recommendations of the committee, RWJF, or the IOM. The section below includes a summary of the remarks that were offered by members of the audience at the forum:

- Several participants described the importance of taking steps to improve the quality of education that students receive. One participant said that to ensure the best possible educational outcomes, quality improvement processes should be applied to nursing education just as they are being applied to the health care system. Another said that nursing education should be evidence-based just as nursing practice should be, and one participant called for federal funding, with more rapid funding cycles, to launch large-scale demonstration projects that can be used to test new educational models. Other participants described a variety of innovative models currently being used that incorporate simulation, technology, residency programs, leadership training, and interdisciplinary education—all of which are designed to better educate nurses.

- One participant highlighted a variety of innovative approaches to education that are being used locally to improve education at the University of Texas Health Science Center at Houston. For example, one model features a bachelor's degree program with clinical immersion; another model includes a regional partnership program with schools and hospitals that use a 100 percent preceptor model. The participant also highlighted a program that features retired physicians who work with nursing students; the participant said that physicians retired from clinical practice have much to teach students about not only clinical skills, but also communicating with physicians.
- A number of participants offered their perspectives on the certification and accreditation of nursing education programs. One participant said that nationwide certification for nursing programs could establish quality expectations, consistency markers, and consumer protections. Another said that nationwide certification for D.N.P. programs could help standardize curriculums, while another said that nursing students at every level should graduate from accredited programs.
- Several audience members offered their opinions on associate degree nursing programs and the importance of opportunities for nurses to move into higher degree programs to ensure a well-educated workforce. One person said the A.D.N. should be a starting point for nursing education, and not an end point; another concurred, highlighting the importance of academic progression to baccalaureate degrees and beyond to master's and doctoral degrees. Another person said that surveys show that most A.D.N.s would like to continue their education. However, a number of barriers, financial and otherwise, keep them from continuing; the participant said these barriers need to be studied so they can be overcome.
- A few participants commented on the importance of partnerships in advancing nursing education. One person said the business community and employers of nurses should be partners in establishing strategic plans for nursing education. Another said that regional partnerships among schools of nursing are required to establish seamless transitions for moving students to higher degree programs, create life-long learners, and help fill nursing

shortages. Another participant described sustained learning communities of students and faculty in partnership with health care agencies and institutes as an example of a seamless learning system that would better represent the real world, while facilitating student movement across care settings.

- One member of the audience highlighted accelerated Ph.D. programs as a possible solution to help alleviate faculty shortages.
- One participant emphasized the need for additional nursing research and funding to support this research. The participant said faculty development and educational processes need to be enhanced at the hundreds of universities that are not academic health centers (where much of the research funding is currently focused) because the majority of nurses and other health care providers are educated at these non-academic health center institutions.
- One participant said the nursing community should be broadly defined to include licensed practical nurses, licensed vocational nurses, and other individuals who deliver care in homes and communities.
- As prompted by the committee's call for testimony that described visions for the future of nursing prior to the forum, a number of people shared their specific visions, which included
    o Students learning multicultural perspectives and receiving education in the area of geriatrics, as the U.S. population continues to grow older and diversify.
    o Using nurse-managed clinics to provide sites for the integration of discovery, learning, and engagement and to allow for the design of new, cost-effective, safe, high-quality, and efficient models of care.
    o Establishing national, evidence-based core competencies in pediatric nursing to ensure that children have a competent pediatric nurse no matter where they are treated.
    o Meeting the needs of nursing graduates from other countries who need to be integrated into U.S. health care settings.

A

References

AANP (American Academy of Nurse Practitioners). 2010. *FAQs about nurse practitioners,* http://www.aanp.org/AANPCMS2/AboutAANP/ About+NPs.htm (accessed May 19, 2010).

Armstrong, M., and S. Frueh, eds. 2003. *Telecommunications for nurses: Providing successful distance education and telehealth.* 2nd ed. New York: Springer.

Benner, P., M. Sutphen, V. Leonard, L. Day, and L. S. Shulman. 2009. *Educating nurses: A call for radical transformation.* San Francisco: Jossey-Bass.

Berlin, L. E., and K. R. Sechrist. 2002. The shortage of doctorally prepared nursing faculty: A dire situation. *Nursing Outlook* 50(2):50–56.

Billings, D., and J. Halstead. 2009. *Teaching in nursing: A guide for faculty.* 3rd ed. St. Louis, MO: Saunders Inc.

Buckley, K. M. 2003. Evaluation of classroom-based, web-enhanced, and web-based distance learning nutrition courses for undergraduate nursing. *Journal of Nursing Education* 42(8):367–370.

Buerhaus, P. I., D. O. Staiger, and D. I. Auerbach. 2000. Implications of an aging registered nurse workforce. *JAMA* 283(22):2948–2954.

Cheng, A., V. Nadkarni, A. Donoghue, K. Nelson, J. L. LeFlore, J. Hopkins, M. Patterson, M. Moyer, M. Brett-Fleegler, M. Kleinman, L. Kappus, W. Eppich, M. Adler, S. Kost, G. Stryjewski, S. Min, J. Podraza, J. Loprelato, M. F. Hamilton, K. Stone, J. Reid, J. Anderson, J. Duff, A. Nishisaki, M. Braga, R. Simon, J. Rudolph, and B. Hunt. 2009. *Examining pediatric resuscitation education using simulation and scripting: The EXPRESS pediatric simulation research collaboration.* Poster presentation at the Second International Pediatric Simulation Symposium and Workshop, April 22–23, Florence, Italy.

Childs, J., and S. Sepples. 2006. Clinical teaching by simulation: Lessons learned from a complex patient care scenario. *Nursing Education Perspectives* 27(3):154–158.

Cunningham, P. J. 2010. The growing financial burden of health care: National and state trends, 2001–2006. *Health Affairs (Millwood)* 29(5):1037–1044.

DeNavas-Walt, C., B. D. Proctor, and J. C. Smith. 2009. *Current population reports: Income, poverty, and health insurance coverage in the United States: 2008.* Washington, DC: U.S. Census Bureau.

HRSA (Health Resources and Services Administration). 2006. *The registered nurse population: Findings from the 2004 National Sample Survey of Registered Nurses.* Washington, DC: HRSA.

HRSA. 2009. *The registered nurse population: Initial findings from the 2008 National Sample Survey of Registered Nurses.* Washington, DC: HRSA.

IOM (Institute of Medicine). 2000. *To err is human: Building a safer health system.* Washington, DC: National Academy Press.

IOM. 2003. *Health professions education: A bridge to quality.* Washington, DC: The National Academies Press.

IOM. 2004. *Keeping patients safe: Transforming the work environment of nurses.* Washington, DC: The National Academies Press.

IOM. 2008. *Retooling for an aging America: Building the health care workforce.* Washington, DC: The National Academies Press.

Jeffries, P. R., S. Rew, and J. M. Cramer. 2002. A comparison of student-centered versus traditional methods of teaching basic nursing skills in a learning laboratory. *Nursing Education Perspectives* 23(1):14–19.

Jeffries, P. R., S. Woolf, and B. Linde. 2003. Technology-based vs. traditional instruction: A comparison of two methods for teaching the skill of performing a 12-lead ECG. *Nursing Education Perspectives* 24(2):70–74.

Joint Commission. 2008. Behaviors that undermine a culture of safety. *Sentinel Event Alert* 40 (July 9).

Jones, C. B. 2008. Revisiting nurse turnover costs: Adjusting for inflation. *Journal of Nursing Administration* 38(1):11–18.

Kaiser Family Foundation, *statehealthfacts.org.* 2010. *Health insurance coverage of the total population, states (2007–2008), U.S. (2008),* http://www.statehealthfacts.org/comparetable.jsp?ind=125&cat=3 (accessed May 27, 2010).

NCSBN (National Council of State Boards of Nursing). 2009. *Description of NCSBN's transition to practice model.* Chicago, IL: NCSBN.

NIH (National Institutes of Health) Office of Budget. 2010. *The National Institutes of Health current operating year, fiscal year 2010: Enacted appropriation,* http://officeofbudget.od.nih.gov/cy.html (accessed May 19, 2010).

Pine, R., and K. Tart. 2007. Return on investment: Benefits and challenges of baccalaureate nurse residency program. *Nursing Economics* 25(1):13–18, 39.

PricewaterhouseCoopers' Health Research Institute. 2007. *What works: Healing the healthcare staffing shortage.* New York: PricewaterhouseCoopers.

Rauen, C. A. 2001. Using simulation to teach critical thinking skills: You can't just throw the book at them. *Critical Care Nursing Clinics of North America* 13(1):93–103.

Simonson, M., S. Smaldino, M. Albright, and S. Zvacek. 2000. *Teaching and learning at a distance: Foundations of distance education.* Upper Saddle River, NJ: Prentice Hall.

U.S. Census Bureau. 2009. *National and state population estimates: Table 3. Estimates of resident population change for the United States, regions, states, and Puerto Rico and region and state rankings: July 1, 2008 to July 1, 2009 (NST-EST2009-03),* http://www.census.gov/popest/states/NST-pop-chg.html (accessed May 27, 2010).

U.S. Census Bureau. 2010. *State & county quickfacts: Colorado,* http://quickfacts.census.gov/qfd/states/08000.html (accessed June 3, 2010).

Wills, C. E., and M. Stommel. 2002. Graduate nursing students' precourse and postcourse perceptions and preferences concerning completely web-based courses. *Journal of Nursing Education* 41(5):193–201.

B

Agenda

FORUM ON THE FUTURE OF NURSING: EDUCATION

University of Texas MD Anderson Cancer Center
Cancer Prevention Building, 8th floor
1155 Pressler Street, Houston, TX 77030

February 22, 2010

AGENDA

8:00 am   **Welcomes and Introductions**
Donna E. Shalala, University of Miami
John R. Lumpkin, Robert Wood Johnson
    Foundation
John Mendelsohn, University of Texas MD
    Anderson Cancer Center

8:15 am   **What We Should Teach: Armchair**
Discussion #1
Moderator: *Michael Bleich, Oregon Health &*
    Science University
Participants:
Linda Cronenwett, University of North
    Carolina–Chapel Hill, School of Nursing

M. Elaine Tagliareni, National League for
    Nursing, formerly Community College of
    Philadelphia
Terry Fulmer, College of Nursing, New York
    University
Marla Salmon, University of Washington School
    of Nursing

9:15 am   **Preselected Testimony**
                     Facilitator: Donna E. Shalala

9:30 am   **How We Should Teach: Armchair**
                     Discussion #2
                     Moderator: Linda Burnes Bolton, Cedars-Sinai
                         Medical Center
                     Participants:
                     Pamela R. Jeffries, Johns Hopkins University
                     Divina Grossman, Florida International
                         University
                     John A. Rock, Florida International University
                     Robert W. Mendenhall, Western Governors
                         University
                     Cathleen Krsek, University HealthSystem
                         Consortium, UHC/AACN Nurse Residency
                         Program™

10:30 am   **Preselected Testimony**
                     Facilitator: Donna E. Shalala

10:45 am   **Break**

11:00 am   **Where We Should Teach: Armchair**
                     Discussion #3
                     Moderator: Jennie Chin Hansen, AARP
                     Participants:
                     Rose Yuhos, AHEC of Southern Nevada
                     Catherine Rick, Department of Veterans Affairs
                         Nursing Academy
                     Christine A. Tanner, Oregon Health & Science
                         University
                     Willis N. Holcombe, Florida College System

12:00 pm **Preselected Testimony**
Facilitator: *Donna E. Shalala*

12:15 pm **Open Microphone Listening Session: Visions for the Future of Nursing**
Facilitator: *Donna E. Shalala*
Participants in the audience will have an opportunity to make impromptu comments on what they heard throughout the day and what their vision is for the future of nursing.

12:35 pm **Closing Remarks**
Donna E. Shalala

12:40 pm **Forum Adjourns**

C

Speaker Biosketches

Michael Bleich, R.N., Ph.D., M.P.H., FAAN, is dean and Dr. Carol A. Lindeman Distinguished Professor for the School of Nursing at Oregon Health & Science University (OHSU). His areas of expertise include leadership development, strategic and operational positioning of academic clinical enterprises, clinical systems design (notably in safety net clinics), work analysis, and quality improvement and outcomes metrics to enhance practice and meet regulatory demands. Dr. Bleich launched his health care career in 1970 and has progressed to hold administrative, education, and consultative roles to the present. He arrived in Portland, Oregon, in 2008, concluding a distinguished career at the University of Kansas, where he was professor and associate dean for Clinical and Community Affairs in the School of Nursing, and concurrently served as executive director/chief executive officer (CEO) of its faculty practice plan, KU HealthPartners, Inc. In 2006, he was appointed chair of the Department of Health Policy and Management in the School of Medicine, the first nurse to hold a chair role.

Linda Burnes Bolton, Dr.P.H., R.N., FAAN, is vice chair, Robert Wood Johnson Foundation (RWJF) Initiative on the Future of Nursing, at the Institute of Medicine (IOM). Dr. Burnes Bolton is vice president for nursing, chief nursing officer, and director of nursing research at Cedars-Sinai Medical Center in Los Angeles. She is one of the principal investigators at the Cedars-Sinai Burns and Allen Research Institute. Her research, teaching, and clinical expertise includes nursing and patient care outcomes research, performance improvement, and improvements in the quality of care and cultural diversity within the health professions. She served as the National Advisory Chair for Transforming Care at the

Bedside, an RWJF initiative, to improve the nursing practice environment. Dr. Burnes Bolton is a past president of the American Academy of Nursing and the National Black Nurses Association.

Linda Cronenwett, Ph.D., R.N., FAAN, is professor and dean emeritus for the School of Nursing at the University of North Carolina–Chapel Hill. Since 2005, she has been the principal investigator of a national initiative, Quality and Safety Education for Nurses, funded by RWJF. Dr. Cronenwett recently cochaired the Josiah Macy Foundation 2010 Conference on Who Should Deliver Primary Care and How Should They Be Trained? She is a current member of the board of directors of the Institute for Healthcare Improvement, the North Carolina Institute of Medicine, and the North Carolina Center for Hospital Quality and Patient Safety. She is also an appointed member of the national Special Medical Advisory Group on Veterans Affairs. Dr. Cronenwett has served as a member of the National Advisory Council for Nursing Research at the National Institutes of Health and in numerous offices in professional associations, including president of the New Hampshire Nurses Association, chair of the American Nurses Association's Congress of Nursing Practice, and chair of the Steering Committee that founded the Eastern Nursing Research Society.

Terry Fulmer, Ph.D., R.N., FAAN, is Erline Perkins McGriff Professor and dean of the College of Nursing at New York University (NYU). Dr. Fulmer joined the NYU faculty in 1995. She is a member of the Executive Committee for the new medical school curriculum and serves as an attending in nursing at the NYU Langone Medical Center. She is a codirector of the John A. Hartford Foundation Institute for Geriatric Nursing and codirector of the Consortium of New York Geriatric Education Centers at NYU. She has spearheaded a number of innovative initiatives at the College of Dentistry at NYU and serves as a member of the Santa Fe Group, a think tank that seeks to identify and implement effective solutions to significant problems in oral health and health care. She has also served on previous panels with the IOM, including Violence in Families: Understanding Prevention and Treatment (1998); Abuse, Neglect, and Exploitation in an Aging America (2003); and Retooling for an Aging America: Building the Health Care Workforce (2007–2008). Dr. Fulmer's program of research focuses on acute care of the elderly, specifically elder abuse and neglect. Dr. Fulmer was the first nurse to be elected to the board of the American Geriatrics Society and the first nurse to serve as president of the Gerontological Society of America.

Divina Grossman, Ph.D., R.N., A.R.N.P., FAAN, was dean of the College of Nursing and Health Sciences at Florida International University (FIU) until her appointment in February 2010 as the founding vice president of engagement at FIU. In this role, Dr. Grossman provides leadership in the development and coordination of focused win–win partnerships with key local, state, national, and global stakeholders. She will also spearhead a university-wide effort to coordinate and expand internship opportunities for undergraduate and graduate students who seek practical experience to augment their formal educations. Additionally, she will have major responsibility for coordinating FIU's effort to receive the Community Engagement classification by the Carnegie Foundation for the Advancement for Teaching. Dr. Grossman began her career as a rural health nurse and a medical–surgical staff nurse, later becoming an assistant professor, department chair for Adult and Gerontological Nursing at FIU, and later department chair for Chronic Nursing Care at the University of Texas Health Sciences Center at San Antonio. She is a clinical specialist in Medical Surgical Nursing and is a licensed Advanced Registered Nurse Practitioner in Florida. Dr. Grossman was the immediate past chair of the American Academy of Nursing's Health Disparities Task Force and cochaired the Academy's national health disparities project funded by the W.K. Kellogg Foundation. At present, she serves as a member of the National Advisory Council of the RWJF's Nurse Faculty Scholars Program, chair of the Florida Association of Colleges of Nursing, board chair of the Kendall Regional Medical Center in Miami, and vice chair of the board of directors of the Health Foundation of South Florida.

Jennie Chin Hansen, R.N., M.S., FAAN, was elected by the AARP board to serve as president for the 2008–2010 biennium. She has previously chaired the board of the AARP Foundation. Ms. Hansen currently holds an appointment as senior fellow at the University of California, San Francisco's Center for the Health Professions and consults with various foundations. She transitioned to teaching in 2005 after nearly 25 years at On Lok, Inc., most recently as its executive director for the last 11 years. On Lok, Inc., is a nonprofit family of organizations providing integrated and comprehensive primary and long-term care community-based services in San Francisco. Ms. Hansen serves in various leadership roles that include commissioner of the Medicare Payment Advisory Commission (MedPAC), and board officer of the National Academy of Social Insurance, the SCAN Foundation, and the Robert Wood Johnson Foundation Executive Nurse Fellows Program. She is also a past president of the American Society on Aging. In April 2010, she became the CEO of the American Geriatrics Society.

Willis N. Holcombe, Ph.D., has been chancellor of Florida College System (formerly the Florida Community College System) since October 2007. The Florida College System is the primary access point to higher education in the state and will serve some 900,000 students this academic year. One of Dr. Holcombe's highest priorities is facilitating and maintaining postsecondary opportunities for Florida students while helping the state's economy recover by enhancing employment related education. He has more than 30 years of experience in educational leadership and collegiate administration, including 17 years as president of Broward Community College. He has also served as vice president of Brevard Community College. Dr. Holcombe has held a vast array of leadership roles and is a highly sought-after speaker, presenter, and consultant to colleges throughout the country. A former U.S. Marine, Dr. Holcombe completed his undergraduate studies at Baldwin-Wallace College and earned both his master's in education and Ph.D. in college administration from the University of Florida.

Pamela R. Jeffries, D.N.S., R.N., FAAN, ANEF, is associate dean of academic affairs at Johns Hopkins University School of Nursing. She has more than 25 years of teaching experience in the classroom, learning laboratory, and clinical setting with undergraduate nursing students. Dr. Jeffries was named project director of the 3-year National League for Nursing (NLN)/Laerdal Simulation Study, a national multisite research project. The overarching purpose of the exploratory, national multisite project was to study various parameters related to the use of simulation in basic nursing education programs and selected student outcomes. She also served as project director for a second NLN/Laerdal grant focused on faculty development for designing and implementing simulations. Nine Web-based courses have been designed and marketed for this project in addition to a global simulation website called the Simulation Innovation Resource Center, which contains many resources for simulation educators. Dr. Jeffries served as principal investigator on an American Heart Association grant to study advanced cardiac life support (ACLS) instruction using high-fidelity manikins. She is currently codirector on a 5-year Health Resources and Services Administration grant directed toward faculty development to teach nurse educators about emerging technologies. Most recently, she is serving as principal investigator for a Who Will Care grant provided by the Maryland Hospital Association that focuses on a new clinical redesign, integration of clinical simulations into the nursing curriculums, and promotion of online course development.

Cathleen Krsek, R.N., M.S.N., M.B.A., is a registered nurse with a clinical background primarily in adult coronary critical care. She has worked in education and quality improvement and has served as a director of nursing. She is currently director of quality operations with the University HealthSystem Consortium, overseeing the Imperatives for Quality program, a new performance improvement approach designed to ensure that academic medical center members demonstrate and are recognized for their leadership in quality, safety, and cost-effectiveness.

John R. Lumpkin, M.D., M.P.H., is senior vice president and director of the Health Care Group at the Robert Wood Johnson Foundation. Before joining the Foundation in April 2003, Dr. Lumpkin served as director of the Illinois Department of Public Health for 12 years. Lumpkin is a member of the IOM and a fellow of the American College of Emergency Physicians and the American College of Medical Informatics. He has been chairman of the National Committee on Vital and Health Statistics, and served on the Council on Maternal, Infant, and Fetal Nutrition, the Advisory Committee to the Director of the U.S. Centers for Disease Control and Prevention, and the IOM's Committee on Assuring the Health of the Public in the 21st Century. Lumpkin has received the Arthur McCormack Excellence and Dedication in Public Health Award from the Association of State and Territorial Health Officials (ASTHO), the Jonas Salk Health Leadership Award, and the Leadership in Public Health Award from the Illinois Public Health Association.

John Mendelsohn, M.D., combines experience in clinical care and research with administrative expertise for leading the University of Texas MD Anderson Cancer Center. Since becoming president in 1996, he has recruited a visionary management team and implemented new priorities for integrated programs in patient care, research, education, and cancer prevention. He has served as founding director of a National Cancer

Institute-designated cancer center at the University of California, San Diego and chair of medicine at Memorial Sloan-Kettering Cancer Center in New York. He and his colleagues pioneered landmark research into EGF receptor blockade as a targeted cancer therapy, which led to the approval of a new cancer drug, Erbitux, and helped launch a productive new field of cancer research. A member of the Institute of Medicine of the National Academy of Sciences, he has received numerous awards and honors, including the Dan David Prize in Cancer Therapy, the Dorothy P. Landon–AACR Prize for Translational Research, and the David A. Karnofsky Memorial Award from the American Society of Clinical Oncology. Under his direction, MD Anderson has been named the top cancer hospital in the nation 6 out of the past 8 years in *U.S. News & World Report*'s "America's Best Hospitals" survey. He has authored more than 300 scientific papers, articles, and chapters, and was the founding editor of the journal *Clinical Cancer Research*. Dr. Mendelsohn serves on numerous community boards, including the Greater Houston Partnership, BioHouston, the Center for Houston's Future, and the Houston Grand Opera. Dr. Mendelsohn is a graduate of Harvard College and Harvard Medical School and recipient of a Fulbright Scholarship to Scotland.

Robert W. Mendenhall, Ph.D., is president of Western Governors University (WGU), a private, not-for-profit, online university offering competency-based bachelor's and master's degrees in business, information technology, K–12 teacher education, and health care (including nursing). The university has 17,000 students in all 50 states and continues to grow at more than 30 percent annually. Dr. Mendenhall has more than 30 years of experience in the development, marketing, and delivery of technology-based education. Prior to WGU, he was general manager of IBM's K–12 education division, overseeing a $500 million worldwide business. From 1980 to 1992, he was a founder, president, and CEO (since 1987) of Wicat Systems, Inc., a publicly traded company that was a leader in computer-based curriculum, instructional management, and testing. Dr. Mendenhall served on the Spellings Commission on the Future of Higher Education, and is a former member of the Utah Board of the Department of Business and Economic Development.

Catherine (Cathy) Rick, R.N., NEA-BC, FACHE, is the chief nursing officer for the Department of Veterans Affairs (VA). Ms. Rick provides leadership and guidance to the VA's 75,000 nursing personnel, who care for more than 5 million veterans a year. As the chief nurse executive for the VA, she is responsible for the development, implementation, and evaluation of national policy and strategic planning activities that support the missions of the Veterans Health Administration: clinical care, education, research, back-up to the Department of Defense, and emergency preparedness. Ms. Rick is responsible for administering the VA National Nursing Strategic Plan. National goals include strategies to enhance leadership excellence, evidence-based practice, informatics, career development and workforce, nursing practice transformation, nursing research, advanced practice nursing, and collaboration with academic affiliates and professional organizations. Significant accomplishments and future directions for each of the goals have emerged. Nursing staff members across the 1,300 VA sites have been affected positively by the work related to these three strategic goals.

John A. Rock, M.D., is senior vice president for medical affairs and founding dean of the Herbert Wertheim College of Medicine at Florida International University. Throughout his career he has brought academic programs to new levels of excellence, increased research productivity, established outstanding patient care units, and fostered excellent educational programs. Dr. Rock is recognized as an outstanding reconstructive surgeon, and his basic research focuses on the pathophysiology of endometriosis and the determination of efficacy of surgical reconstructive procedures and medical therapy using the randomized clinical trial. He was the first to recognize and describe the presence of microscopic endometriosis, which was the basis of the introduction of new therapies for this complex disease. He has published extensively on the diagnosis and treatment of uterovaginal anomalies, and his surgical innovations have improved the reproductive outcomes of these disorders. He is the senior editor of *Telinde's Operative Gynecology*, one of the most respected textbooks in the field of gynecologic surgery. He has served as president of the Society of Gynecologic Surgeons, the American Society for Reproductive Medicine, and the World Endometriosis Society.

Marla Salmon, Sc.D., R.N., FAAN, is Robert G. and Jean A. Reid Endowed Dean in Nursing and professor in the School of Nursing at the University of Washington (UW). She is also a professor in UW's Department of Global Health. Her experience includes directing the Division of Nursing for the U.S. Department of Health and Human Services (HHS) and chairing the Global Advisory Group on Nursing and Midwifery for the World Health Organization and the National Advisory Committee on Nursing Education and Practice. She founded and directed the Lillian Carter Center for International Nursing and is a director on the RWJF Board of Trustees, a member of the National Advisory Council for Nursing Research, and a director for the Institute for the International Education of Students. Her scholarship focuses on global and domestic health workforce policy and leadership. She consults with governments and regional and global organizations.

Donna E. Shalala, Ph.D., FAAN, is chair of the RWJF Initiative on the Future of Nursing at the IOM. She is president of the University of Miami and a professor of political science. She has more than 25 years of experience as an accomplished scholar, teacher, and administrator. A leading scholar on the political economy of state and local governments, she has also held tenured professorships at Columbia University, the City University of New York (CUNY), and the University of Wisconsin–Madison. She served as president of CUNY's Hunter College from 1980 to 1987 and as chancellor of the University of Wisconsin–Madison from 1987 to 1993. In 1993, President Bill Clinton appointed her as Secretary of Health and Human Services, where she served for 8 years, becoming the longest serving HHS Secretary in U.S. history.

M. Elaine Tagliareni, Ed.D., R.N., C.N.E., FAAN, is chief program officer for the National League for Nursing. In this position she advocates for excellence in nursing education through pedagogical research and initiates faculty development strategies to prepare a strong, competent, and diverse nursing workforce. Prior to this appointment in January 2010, Dr. Tagliareni was a professor of nursing and the Independence Foundation Chair in Community Health Nursing Education at Community College of Philadelphia, where she served as an associate degree nursing educator for more than 25 years. She received her B.S.N. from Georgetown University School of Nursing, a master's in Mental Health and Community Nursing from the University of California–San Francisco, and a doctorate from Teachers College, Columbia University, with an emphasis on the role of the nurse educator in community colleges.

Christine A. Tanner, R.N., Ph.D., FAAN, is A.B. Youmans-Spaulding Distinguished Professor at OHSU and editor-in-chief of the *Journal of Nursing Education.* Dr. Tanner's program of research focuses on development of expertise in clinical judgment and the impact of different education models on the development of skill in clinical judgment. For the past decade, she has been one of Oregon's leaders in creating educational solutions to the nursing shortage, including ways to increase enrollment and prepare a new kind of nurse in the context of rapid changes in the nursing practice environment and health care needs. The Oregon Consortium for Nursing Education (OCNE) was launched in 2003 as a partnership among OHSU and several community colleges. It is designed to incorporate best practices in teaching and learning with a shared curriculum that focuses on care-health promotion, chronic illness management, acute care, and skills needed by the nurse in this rapidly changing environment. This environment includes population-based and systems thinking, sound clinical judgment using best available evidence, and the ability to work with and lead interdisciplinary teams. Dr. Tanner is currently principal investigator for two studies: one focused on evaluating the outcomes of OCNE, and the second on the effectiveness of a new clinical education model designed, in part, to increase educational capacity.

Rose Yuhos, R.N., has been executive director of the Area Health Education Center (AHEC) of Southern Nevada for the past 19 years. This nonprofit organization provides continuing education for health care professionals; enrichment and health career awareness programs, as well academic areas for at-risk students; family and life skills training; and outreach for women who need screening and treatment for breast and cervical cancer. In this role, Ms. Yuhos provides leadership, grant direction, and management of all aspects of AHEC programs. She develops community outreach, staff supervision, and fiscal management of professional education curriculums, and serves as ex-officio member of the AHEC Board of Trustees. Prior to her current position, Ms. Yuhos served as associate director of the Las Vegas AIDS Education and Training Center; director of clinical services for the Community Health Centers of Southern Nevada; and program specialist for AHEC of Southern Nevada.